Cram101 Textbook Outlines to accompany:

Healthcare Finance: An Introduction To Accounting And Financial Management

Gapenski, 3rd Edition

An Academic Internet Publishers (AIPI) publication (c) 2007.

Cram101 and Cram101.com are AIPI publications and services. All notes, highlights, reviews, and practice tests are prepared by AIPI for use in AIPI publications, all rights reserved.

You have a discounted membership at www.Cram101.com with this book.

Get all of the practice tests for the chapters of this textbook, and access in-depth reference material for writing essays and papers. Here is an example from a Cram101 Biology text:

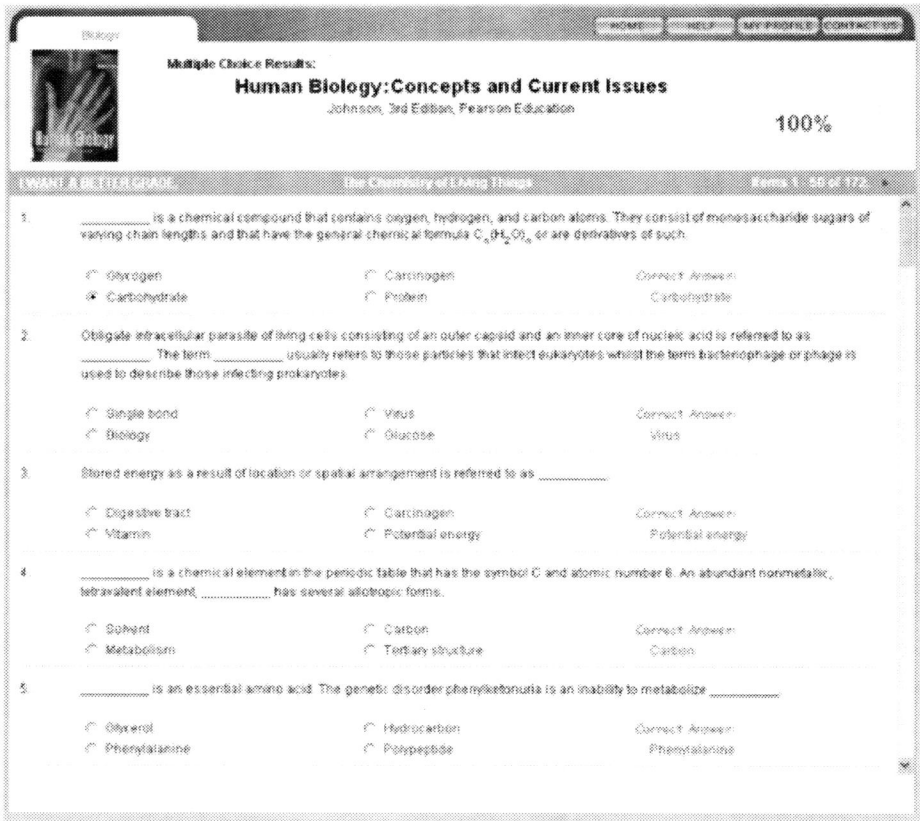

When you need problem solving help with math, stats, and other disciplines, www.Cram101.com will walk through the formulas and solutions step by step.

With Cram101.com online, you also have access to extensive reference material.

You will nail those essays and papers. Here is an example from a Cram101 Biology text:

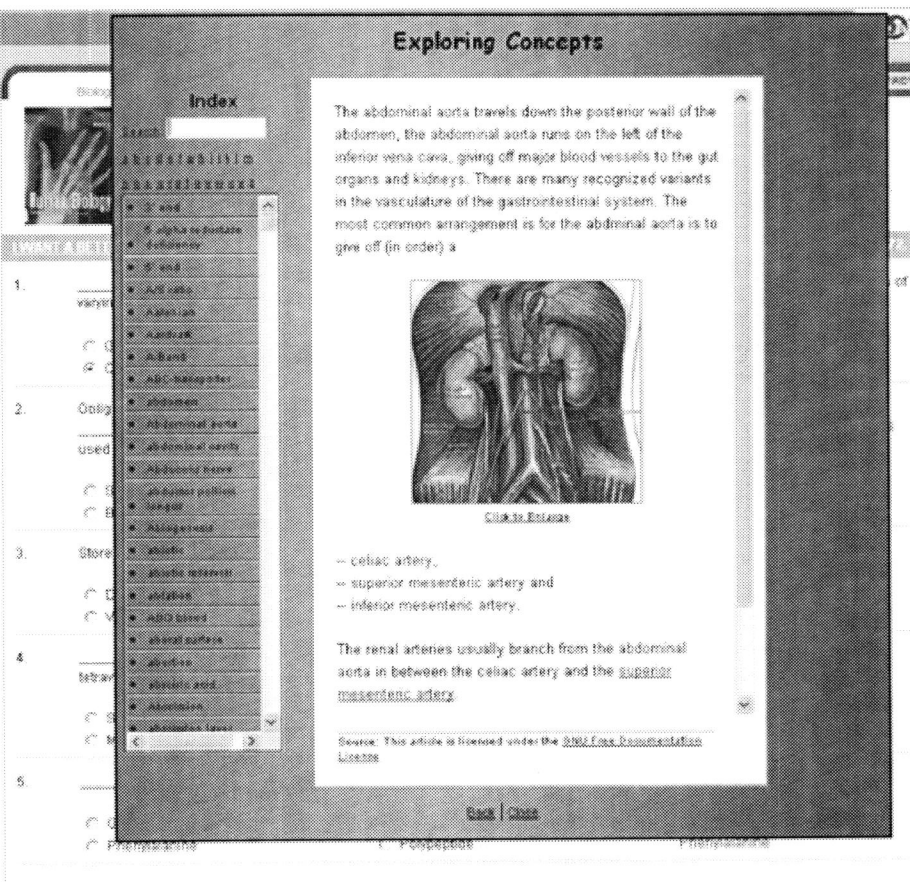

Visit **www.Cram101.com**, click Sign Up at the top of the screen, and enter DK73DW3544 in the promo code box on the registration screen. Access to www.Cram101.com is normally $9.95, but because you have purchased this book, your access fee is only $4.95. Sign up and stop highlighting textbooks forever.

Learning System

Cram101 Textbook Outlines is a learning system. The notes in this book are the highlights of your textbook, you will never have to highlight a book again.

How to use this book. Take this book to class, it is your notebook for the lecture. The notes and highlights on the left hand side of the pages follow the outline and order of the textbook. All you have to do is follow along while your intructor presents the lecture. Circle the items emphasized in class and add other important information on the right side. With Cram101 Textbook Outlines you'll spend less time writing and more time listening. Learning becomes more efficient.

Cram101.com Online

Increase your studying efficiency by using Cram101.com's practice tests and online reference material. It is the perfect complement to Cram101 Textbook Outlines. Use self-teaching matching tests or simulate in-class testing with comprehensive multiple choice tests, or simply use Cram's true and false tests for quick review. Cram101.com even allows you to enter your in-class notes for an integrated studying format combining the textbook notes with your class notes.

Visit **www.Cram101.com**, click Sign Up at the top of the screen, and enter **DK73DW3544** in the promo code box on the registration screen. Access to www.Cram101.com is normally $9.95, but because you have purchased this book, your access fee is only $4.95. Sign up and stop highlighting textbooks forever.

Copyright © 2007 by Academic Internet Publishers, Inc. All rights reserved. "Cram101"® and "Never Highlight a Book Again!"® are registered trademarks of Academic Internet Publishers, Inc. The Cram101 Textbook Outline series is printed in the United States. ISBN: 1-4288-1287-3

Healthcare Finance: An Introduction To Accounting And Financial Management
Gapenski, 3rd

CONTENTS

1. Introduction to Healthcare Finance 2
2. The Financial Environment 12
3. Financial Accounting Basics and the Income Statement 30
4. The Balance Sheet and Statement of Cash Flows 50
5. Managerial Accounting Basics, Cost Behavior and Profit Analysis 68
6. Cost Allocation 78
7. Pricing and Service Decisions 86
8. Planning and Budgeting 96
9. Time Value Analysis 110
10. Financial Risk and Required Return 120
11. Long-Term Debt Financing 130
12. Equity Financing 152
13. Capital Structure and the Cost of Capital 172
14. The Basics of Capital Budgeting 190
15. Project Risk Assessment and Incorporation 206
16. Current Asset Management and Financing 218
17. Analyzing Financial Performance 238
18. Lease Financing and Business Valuation 258

Chapter 1. Introduction to Healthcare Finance

Service	Service refers to a "non tangible product" that is not embodied in a physical good and that typically effects some change in another product, person, or institution. Contrasts with good.
Industry	A group of firms that produce identical or similar products is an industry. It is also used specifically to refer to an area of economic production focused on manufacturing which involves large amounts of capital investment before any profit can be realized, also called "heavy industry".
Health insurance	Health insurance is a type of insurance whereby the insurer pays the medical costs of the insured if the insured becomes sick due to covered causes, or due to accidents. The insurer may be a private organization or a government agency.
Insurance	Insurance refers to a system by which individuals can reduce their exposure to risk of large losses by spreading the risks among a large number of persons.
Health maintenance organizations	Health care providers that contract with employers, insurance companies, labor unions, or government units to provide health care for their workers or others who are insured are referred to as health maintenance organizations.
Health maintenance organization	A Health Maintenance Organization is a fixed, prepaid health care plan that provides comprehensive benefits for employees who are required to use a network of participating providers for all health services.
Accounting	A system that collects and processes financial information about an organization and reports that information to decision makers is referred to as accounting.
Operation	A standardized method or technique that is performed repetitively, often on different materials resulting in different finished goods is called an operation.
Context	The effect of the background under which a message often takes on more and richer meaning is a context. Context is especially important in cross-cultural interactions because some cultures are said to be high context or low context.
Enterprise	Enterprise refers to another name for a business organization. Other similar terms are business firm, sometimes simply business, sometimes simply firm, as well as company, and entity.
Financial management	The job of managing a firm's resources so it can meet its goals and objectives is called financial management.
Management	Management characterizes the process of leading and directing all or part of an organization, often a business, through the deployment and manipulation of resources. Early twentieth-century management writer Mary Parker Follett defined management as "the art of getting things done through people."
Chief financial officer	Chief financial officer refers to executive responsible for overseeing the financial operations of an organization.
Senior management	Senior management is generally a team of individuals at the highest level of organizational management who have the day-to-day responsibilities of managing a corporation.
Investment	Investment refers to spending for the production and accumulation of capital and additions to inventories. In a financial sense, buying an asset with the expectation of making a return.
Capital	Capital generally refers to financial wealth, especially that used to start or maintain a business. In classical economics, capital is one of four factors of production, the others being land and labor and entrepreneurship.
Asset	An item of property, such as land, capital, money, a share in ownership, or a claim on others for future payment, such as a bond or a bank deposit is an asset.
Inventory	Tangible property held for sale in the normal course of business or used in producing goods or services for sale is an inventory.
Security	Security refers to a claim on the borrower future income that is sold by the borrower to the lender. A

Chapter 1. Introduction to Healthcare Finance

Chapter 1. Introduction to Healthcare Finance

security is a type of transferable interest representing financial value.

Marketable securities	Marketable securities refer to securities that are readily traded in the secondary securities market.
Working capital management	Working capital management refers to the financing and management of the current assets of the firm. The financial manager determines the mix between temporary and permanent 'current assets' and the nature of the financing arrangement.
Asset management	Asset management is the method that a company uses to track fixed assets, for example factory equipment, desks and chairs, computers, even buildings. Although the exact details of the task varies widely from company to company, asset management often includes tracking the physical location of assets, managing demand for scarce resources, and accounting tasks such as amortization.
Working capital	The dollar difference between total current assets and total current liabilities is called working capital.
Contract	A contract is a "promise" or an "agreement" that is enforced or recognized by the law. In the civil law, a contract is considered to be part of the general law of obligations.
Financial transaction	A financial transaction involves a change in the status of the finances of two or more businesses or individuals.
Cost accounting	Cost accounting measures and reports financial and nonfinancial information relating to the cost of acquiring or consuming resources in an organization. It provides information for both management accounting and financial accounting.
Regulation	Regulation refers to restrictions state and federal laws place on business with regard to the conduct of its activities.
Medicare	Medicare refers to federal program that is financed by payroll taxes and provides for compulsory hospital insurance for senior citizens and low-cost voluntary insurance to help older Americans pay physicians' fees.
Revenue	Revenue is a U.S. business term for the amount of money that a company receives from its activities, mostly from sales of products and/or services to customers.
Complexity	The technical sophistication of the product and hence the amount of understanding required to use it is referred to as complexity. It is the opposite of simplicity.
Joint venture	Joint venture refers to an undertaking by two parties for a specific purpose and duration, taking any of several legal forms.
Negotiation	Negotiation is the process whereby interested parties resolve disputes, agree upon courses of action, bargain for individual or collective advantage, and/or attempt to craft outcomes which serve their mutual interests.
Human resource management	The process of evaluating human resource needs, finding people to fill those needs, and getting the best work from each employee by providing the right incentives and job environment, all with the goal of meeting the needs of the firm are called human resource management.
Resource management	Resource management is the efficient and effective deployment of an organization's resources when they are needed. Such resources may include financial resources, inventory, human skills, production resources, or information technology.
Senior executive	Senior executive means a chief executive officer, chief operating officer, chief financial officer and anyone in charge of a principal business unit or function.
Marketing	Promoting and selling products or services to customers, or prospective customers, is referred to as marketing.
Ambulatory care	Ambulatory care is any medical care delivered on an outpatient basis. Many medical conditions do not

Chapter 1. Introduction to Healthcare Finance

Chapter 1. Introduction to Healthcare Finance

	require hospital admission and can be managed without admission to a hospital. Many medical investigations can be performed on an ambulatory basis, including blood tests, X-rays, endoscopy and even biopsy procedures of superficial organs.
Compliance	A type of influence process where a receiver accepts the position advocated by a source to obtain favorable outcomes or to avoid punishment is the compliance.
Fund	Independent accounting entity with a self-balancing set of accounts segregated for the purposes of carrying on specific activities is referred to as a fund.
Contribution	In business organization law, the cash or property contributed to a business by its owners is referred to as contribution.
Annuities	Financial contracts under which a customer pays an annual premium in exchange for a future stream of annual payments beginning at a set age, say 65, and ending when the person dies are annuities.
Property	Assets defined in the broadest legal sense. Property includes the unrealized receivables of a cash basis taxpayer, but not services rendered.
Annuity	A contract to make regular payments to a person for life or for a fixed period is an annuity.
Charitable contributions	Charitable contributions refers to contributions that are tax deductible if made to qualified nonprofit charitable organizations. A cash basis taxpayer is entitled to a deduction solely in the year of payment.
Corporation	A legal entity chartered by a state or the Federal government that is distinct and separate from the individuals who own it is a corporation. This separation gives the corporation unique powers which other legal entities lack.
Labor	People's physical and mental talents and efforts that are used to help produce goods and services are called labor.
Privilege	Generally, a legal right to engage in conduct that would otherwise result in legal liability is a privilege. Privileges are commonly classified as absolute or conditional. Occasionally, privilege is also used to denote a legal right to refrain from particular behavior.
Petition	A petition is a request to an authority, most commonly a government official or public entity. In the colloquial sense, a petition is a document addressed to some official and signed by numerous individuals.
Ambulatory surgery	Surgery done in the doctor's office or at a surgical center, and not requiring an overnight stay. Ambulatory surgery is general planned ahead of time. Maybe referred to as one-day, in-and-out, or outpatient surgery.
Technology	The body of knowledge and techniques that can be used to combine economic resources to produce goods and services is called technology.
Incentive	An incentive is any factor (financial or non-financial) that provides a motive for a particular course of action, or counts as a reason for preferring one choice to the alternatives.
Continuity	A media scheduling strategy where a continuous pattern of advertising is used over the time span of the advertising campaign is continuity.
Administrator	Administrator refers to the personal representative appointed by a probate court to settle the estate of a deceased person who died.
Intervention	Intervention refers to an activity in which a government buys or sells its currency in the foreign exchange market in order to affect its currency's exchange rate.
Gatekeeper	Gatekeeper refers to an individual who has a strategic position in the network that allows him or her to control information moving in either direction through a channel.

Chapter 1. Introduction to Healthcare Finance

Chapter 1. Introduction to Healthcare Finance

Quality management	Quality management is a method for ensuring that all the activities necessary to design, develop and implement a product or service are effective and efficient with respect to the system and its performance.
Distribution	Distribution in economics, the manner in which total output and income is distributed among individuals or factors.
Gain	In finance, gain is a profit or an increase in value of an investment such as a stock or bond. Gain is calculated by fair market value or the proceeds from the sale of the investment minus the sum of the purchase price and all costs associated with it.
Welfare	Welfare refers to the economic well being of an individual, group, or economy. For individuals, it is conceptualized by a utility function. For groups, including countries and the world, it is a tricky philosophical concept, since individuals fare differently.
Extension	Extension refers to an out-of-court settlement in which creditors agree to allow the firm more time to meet its financial obligations. A new repayment schedule will be developed, subject to the acceptance of creditors.
Capital expenditures	Major investments in long-term assets such as land, buildings, equipment, or research and development are referred to as capital expenditures.
Capital expenditure	A substantial expenditure that is used by a company to acquire or upgrade physical assets such as equipment, property, industrial buildings, including those which improve the quality and life of an asset is referred to as a capital expenditure.
Administrative cost	An administrative cost is all executive, organizational, and clerical costs associated with the general management of an organization rather than with manufacturing, marketing, or selling
Inflation	An increase in the overall price level of an economy, usually as measured by the CPI or by the implicit price deflator is called inflation.
Budget	Budget refers to an account, usually for a year, of the planned expenditures and the expected receipts of an entity. For a government, the receipts are tax revenues.
Regulatory agency	Regulatory agency refers to an agency, commission, or board established by the Federal government or a state government to regulates businesses in the public interest.
Liability	A liability is a present obligation of the enterprise arizing from past events, the settlement of which is expected to result in an outflow from the enterprise of resources embodying economic benefits.
Quality assurance	Those activities associated with assuring the quality of a product or service is called quality assurance.
Premium	Premium refers to the fee charged by an insurance company for an insurance policy. The rate of losses must be relatively predictable: In order to set the premium (prices) insurers must be able to estimate them accurately.
Litigation	The process of bringing, maintaining, and defending a lawsuit is litigation.
Tort	In the common law, a tort is a civil wrong, other than a breach of contract, for which the law provides a remedy. A tort is a breach of a non-contractual duty potentially owed to the entire world, imposed by law. The majority of legal claims are brought in tort.
Antitrust	Government intervention to alter market structure or prevent abuse of market power is called antitrust.
Financial accounting	Financial accounting is the branch of accountancy concerned with the preparation of financial statements for external decision makers, such as stockholders, suppliers, banks and government agencies. The fundamental need for financial accounting is to reduce principal-agent problem by measuring and monitoring agents' performance.
Income statement	Income statement refers to a financial statement that presents the revenues and expenses and resulting

Chapter 1. Introduction to Healthcare Finance

Chapter 1. Introduction to Healthcare Finance

	net income or net loss of a company for a specific period of time.
Balance sheet	A statement of the assets, liabilities, and net worth of a firm or individual at some given time often at the end of its "fiscal year," is referred to as a balance sheet.
Cash flow	In finance, cash flow refers to the amounts of cash being received and spent by a business during a defined period of time, sometimes tied to a specific project. Most of the time they are being used to determine gaps in the liquid position of a company.
Balance	In banking and accountancy, the outstanding balance is the amount of money owned, (or due), that remains in a deposit account (or a loan account) at a given date, after all past remittances, payments and withdrawal have been accounted for. It can be positive (then, in the balance sheet of a firm, it is an asset) or negative (a liability).
Statement of cash flow	Reports inflows and outflows of cash during the accounting period in the categories of operating, investing, and financing is a statement of cash flow.
Cost allocation	Cost allocation refers to the process of assigning costs in a cost pool to the appropriate cost objects.
Cost behavior	The relationship between cost and volume or activity is referred to as cost behavior.
Profit	Profit refers to the return to the resource entrepreneurial ability; total revenue minus total cost.
Financial analysis	Financial analysis is the analysis of the accounts and the economic prospects of a firm.
Acquisition	A company's purchase of the property and obligations of another company is an acquisition.
Capital budgeting	Capital budgeting is the planning process used to determine a firm's long term investments such as new machinery, replacement machinery, new plants, new products, and research and development projects.
Aid	Assistance provided by countries and by international institutions such as the World Bank to developing countries in the form of monetary grants, loans at low interest rates, in kind, or a combination of these is called aid. Aid can also refer to assistance of any type rendered to benefit some group or individual.
Personnel	A collective term for all of the employees of an organization. Personnel is also commonly used to refer to the personnel management function or the organizational unit responsible for administering personnel programs.
Private sector	The households and business firms of the economy are referred to as private sector.
Controlling	A management function that involves determining whether or not an organization is progressing toward its goals and objectives, and taking corrective action if it is not is called controlling.
Journal	Book of original entry, in which transactions are recorded in a general ledger system, is referred to as a journal.
Administration	Administration refers to the management and direction of the affairs of governments and institutions; a collective term for all policymaking officials of a government; the execution and implementation of public policy.

Chapter 1. Introduction to Healthcare Finance

Chapter 2. The Financial Environment

Incentive	An incentive is any factor (financial or non-financial) that provides a motive for a particular course of action, or counts as a reason for preferring one choice to the alternatives.
Industry	A group of firms that produce identical or similar products is an industry. It is also used specifically to refer to an area of economic production focused on manufacturing which involves large amounts of capital investment before any profit can be realized, also called "heavy industry".
Corporation	A legal entity chartered by a state or the Federal government that is distinct and separate from the individuals who own it is a corporation. This separation gives the corporation unique powers which other legal entities lack.
Financial management	The job of managing a firm's resources so it can meet its goals and objectives is called financial management.
Accounting	A system that collects and processes financial information about an organization and reports that information to decision makers is referred to as accounting.
Management	Management characterizes the process of leading and directing all or part of an organization, often a business, through the deployment and manipulation of resources. Early twentieth-century management writer Mary Parker Follett defined management as "the art of getting things done through people."
Partnership	In the common law, a partnership is a type of business entity in which partners share with each other the profits or losses of the business undertaking in which they have all invested.
Service	Service refers to a "non tangible product" that is not embodied in a physical good and that typically effects some change in another product, person, or institution. Contrasts with good.
Sole proprietorship	A sole proprietorship is a business which legally has no separate existence from its owner. Hence, the limitations of liability enjoyed by a corporation do not apply.
Business operations	Business operations are those activities involved in the running of a business for the purpose of producing value for the stakeholders. The outcome of business operations is the harvesting of value from assets owned by a business.
Operation	A standardized method or technique that is performed repetitively, often on different materials resulting in different finished goods is called an operation.
Regulation	Regulation refers to restrictions state and federal laws place on business with regard to the conduct of its activities.
Corporate level	Corporate level refers to level at which top management directs overall strategy for the entire organization.
Capital gain	Capital gain refers to the gain in value that the owner of an asset experiences when the price of the asset rises, including when the currency in which the asset is denominated appreciates.
Stockholder	A stockholder is an individual or company (including a corporation) that legally owns one or more shares of stock in a joined stock company. The shareholders are the owners of a corporation. Companies listed at the stock market strive to enhance shareholder value.
Dividend	Amount of corporate profits paid out for each share of stock is referred to as dividend.
Capital	Capital generally refers to financial wealth, especially that used to start or maintain a business. In classical economics, capital is one of four factors of production, the others being land and labor and entrepreneurship.

Chapter 2. The Financial Environment

Chapter 2. The Financial Environment

Profit	Profit refers to the return to the resource entrepreneurial ability; total revenue minus total cost.
Gain	In finance, gain is a profit or an increase in value of an investment such as a stock or bond. Gain is calculated by fair market value or the proceeds from the sale of the investment minus the sum of the purchase price and all costs associated with it.
Liability	A liability is a present obligation of the enterprise arizing from past events, the settlement of which is expected to result in an outflow from the enterprise of resources embodying economic benefits.
Unlimited liability	Absence of any limits on the maximum amount that an individual may become legally required to pay is called unlimited liability.
Bankruptcy	Bankruptcy is a legally declared inability or impairment of ability of an individual or organization to pay their creditors.
Pro rata	Proportionate is referred to as pro rata. A method of equally and proportionately allocating money, profits or liabilities by percentage.
Asset	An item of property, such as land, capital, money, a share in ownership, or a claim on others for future payment, such as a bond or a bank deposit is an asset.
Legal entity	A legal entity is a legal construct through which the law allows a group of natural persons to act as if it were an individual for certain purposes. The most common purposes are lawsuits, property ownership, and contracts.
Shares	Shares refer to an equity security, representing a shareholder's ownership of a corporation. Shares are one of a finite number of equal portions in the capital of a company, entitling the owner to a proportion of distributed, non-reinvested profits known as dividends and to a portion of the value of the company in case of liquidation.
Stock	In financial terminology, stock is the capital raized by a corporation, through the issuance and sale of shares.
Charter	Charter refers to an instrument or authority from the sovereign power bestowing the right or power to do business under the corporate form of organization. Also, the organic law of a city or town, and representing a portion of the statute law of the state.
Bylaw	In corporation law, a document that supplements the articles of incorporation and contains less important rights, powers, and responsibilities of a corporation and its shareholders, officers, and directors is referred to as a bylaw.
No frills	No frills is the term used to describe any service or product for which the non-essential features have been removed.
Annual report	An annual report is prepared by corporate management that presents financial information including financial statements, footnotes, and the management discussion and analysis.
Shareholder	A shareholder is an individual or company (including a corporation) that legally owns one or more shares of stock in a joined stock company.
Firm	An organization that employs resources to produce a good or service for profit and owns and operates one or more plants is referred to as a firm.
Investment	Investment refers to spending for the production and accumulation of capital and additions to inventories. In a financial sense, buying an asset with the expectation of making a return.
Liquidity	Liquidity refers to the capacity to turn assets into cash, or the amount of assets in a portfolio that have that capacity.
Equity	Equity investment generally refers to the buying and holding of shares of stock on a stock

Chapter 2. The Financial Environment

Chapter 2. The Financial Environment

investment	market by individuals and funds in anticipation of income from dividends and capital gain as the value of the stock rises.
Equity	Equity is the name given to the set of legal principles, in countries following the English common law tradition, which supplement strict rules of law where their application would operate harshly, so as to achieve what is sometimes referred to as "natural justice."
General partners	Partners in a limited partnership who invest capital, manage the business, and are personally liable for partnership debts are referred to as general partners.
Limited partner	An owner of a limited partnership who has no right to manage the business but who possesses liability limited to his capital contribution to the business is referred to as limited partner.
General partner	An owner who has unlimited liability and is active in managing the firm is a general partner. The individual or firm that organizes and manages the limited partnership. For example a hedge fund.
Limited partnership	A partnership in which some of the partners are limited partners. At least one of the partners in a limited partnership must be a general partner.
Estate	An estate is the totality of the legal rights, interests, entitlements and obligations attaching to property. In the context of wills and probate, it refers to the totality of the property which the deceased owned or in which some interest was held.
Limited liability partnership	Limited liability partnership refers to a form of business organization allowed by many of the states, where partners have a form of limited liability, similar to that of the shareholders of a corporation.
Limited liability	Limited liability is a liability that is limited to a partner or investor's investment. Shareholders in a corporation or in a limited liability company cannot lose more money than the value of their shares if the corporation runs into debt, as they are not personally responsible for the corporation's obligations.
Joint liability	Liability of a group of persons in which, if one of these persons is sued, he can insist that the other liable parties be joined to the suit as codefendants, so that all must be sued collectively is referred to as joint liability.
Limited liability company	Limited liability company refers to a form of entity allowed by all of the states. The entity is taxed as a partnership in which all members or owners of the limited liability company are treated much like limited partners.
Incorporation	Incorporation is the forming of a new corporation. The corporation may be a business, a non-profit organization or even a government of a new city or town.
Statute	A statute is a formal, written law of a country or state, written and enacted by its legislative authority, perhaps to then be ratified by the highest executive in the government, and finally published.
S corporation	One designation for a small business corporation is a S corporation.
Economy	The income, expenditures, and resources that affect the cost of running a business and household are called an economy.
General Electric	In 1876, Thomas Alva Edison opened a new laboratory in Menlo Park, New Jersey. Out of the laboratory was to come perhaps the most famous invention of all—a successful development of the incandescent electric lamp. By 1890, Edison had organized his various businesses into the Edison General Electric Company.
Ford	Ford is an American company that manufactures and sells automobiles worldwide. Ford introduced methods for large-scale manufacturing of cars, and large-scale management of an

Chapter 2. The Financial Environment

Chapter 2. The Financial Environment

	industrial workforce, especially elaborately engineered manufacturing sequences typified by the moving assembly lines.
Common stock	Common stock refers to the basic, normal, voting stock issued by a corporation; called residual equity because it ranks after preferred stock for dividend and liquidation distributions.
Primary market	The market for the raising of new funds as opposed to the trading of securities already in existence is called primary market.
Market	A market is, as defined in economics, a social arrangement that allows buyers and sellers to discover information and carry out a voluntary exchange of goods or services.
Secondary market	Secondary market refers to the market for securities that have already been issued. It is a market in which investors trade back and forth with each other.
Enterprise	Enterprise refers to another name for a business organization. Other similar terms are business firm, sometimes simply business, sometimes simply firm, as well as company, and entity.
Publicly held corporation	Publicly held corporation refers to a corporation that may have thousands of stockholders and whose stock is regularly traded on a national securities market.
Pfizer	Pfizer is the world's largest pharmaceutical company based in New York City. It produces the number-one selling drug Lipitor (atorvastatin, used to lower blood cholesterol).
Privately held corporation	A corporation that has only a few stockholders and whose stock is not available for sale to the general public is a privately held corporation.
Board of directors	The group of individuals elected by the stockholders of a corporation to oversee its operations is a board of directors.
Common stockholder	A person who owns common stock is referred to as common stockholder. They elect the members of the board of directors for the company, as well.
Proxy	Proxy refers to a person who is authorized to vote the shares of another person. Also, the written authorization empowering a person to vote the shares of another person.
Revenue	Revenue is a U.S. business term for the amount of money that a company receives from its activities, mostly from sales of products and/or services to customers.
Debt capital	Debt capital refers to funds raized through various forms of borrowing to finance a company that must be repaid.
Insurance	Insurance refers to a system by which individuals can reduce their exposure to risk of large losses by spreading the risks among a large number of persons.
Expense	In accounting, an expense represents an event in which an asset is used up or a liability is incurred. In terms of the accounting equation, expenses reduce owners' equity.
Labor	People's physical and mental talents and efforts that are used to help produce goods and services are called labor.
Residual	Residual payments can refer to an ongoing stream of payments in respect of the completion of past achievements.
Liquidation	Liquidation refers to a process whereby the assets of a business are converted to money. The conversion may be coerced by a legal process to pay off the debt of the business, or to satisfy any other business obligation that the business has not voluntarily satisfied.
Internal Revenue Service	In 1862, during the Civil War, President Lincoln and Congress created the office of Commissioner of Internal Revenue and enacted an income tax to pay war expenses. The position

Chapter 2. The Financial Environment

Chapter 2. The Financial Environment

of Commissioner still exists today. The Commissioner is the head of the Internal Revenue Service.

Foundation	A Foundation is a type of philanthropic organization set up by either individuals or institutions as a legal entity (either as a corporation or trust) with the purpose of distributing grants to support causes in line with the goals of the foundation.
Fund	Independent accounting entity with a self-balancing set of accounts segregated for the purposes of carrying on specific activities is referred to as a fund.
Promotion	Promotion refers to all the techniques sellers use to motivate people to buy products or services. An attempt by marketers to inform people about products and to persuade them to participate in an exchange.
Interest	In finance and economics, interest is the price paid by a borrower for the use of a lender's money. In other words, interest is the amount of paid to "rent" money for a period of time.
Federal government	Federal government refers to the government of the United States, as distinct from the state and local governments.
Organizational goals	Objectives that management seeks to achieve in pursuing the firm's purpose are organizational goals.
Equity financing	Financing that consists of funds that are invested in exchange for ownership in the company is called equity financing.
Security	Security refers to a claim on the borrower future income that is sold by the borrower to the lender. A security is a type of transferable interest representing financial value.
Small business	Small business refers to a business that is independently owned and operated, is not dominant in its field of operation, and meets certain standards of size in terms of employees or annual receipts.
Welfare	Welfare refers to the economic well being of an individual, group, or economy. For individuals, it is conceptualized by a utility function. For groups, including countries and the world, it is a tricky philosophical concept, since individuals fare differently.
Shareholder wealth maximization	Shareholder wealth maximization refers to maximizing the wealth of the firm's shareholders through achieving the highest possible value for the firm in the marketplace. It is the overriding objective of the firm and should influence all decisions.
Principal	In agency law, one under whose direction an agent acts and for whose benefit that agent acts is a principal.
Authority	Authority in agency law, refers to an agent's ability to affect his principal's legal relations with third parties. Also used to refer to an actor's legal power or ability to do something. In addition, sometimes used to refer to a statute, case, or other legal source that justifies a particular result.
Agent	A person who makes economic decisions for another economic actor. A hired manager operates as an agent for a firm's owner.
Stock option	A stock option is a specific type of option that uses the stock itself as an underlying instrument to determine the option's pay-off and therefore its value.
Option	A contract that gives the purchaser the option to buy or sell the underlying financial instrument at a specified price, called the exercise price or strike price, within a specific period of time.
Stakeholder	A stakeholder is an individual or group with a vested interest in or expectation for organizational performance. Usually stakeholders can either have an effect on or are affected

Chapter 2. The Financial Environment

Chapter 2. The Financial Environment

	by an organization.
Mission statement	Mission statement refers to an outline of the fundamental purposes of an organization.
Technology	The body of knowledge and techniques that can be used to combine economic resources to produce goods and services is called technology.
Grant	Grant refers to an intergovernmental transfer of funds . Since the New Deal, state and local governments have become increasingly dependent upon federal grants for an almost infinite variety of programs.
Long run	In economic models, the long run time frame assumes no fixed factors of production. Firms can enter or leave the marketplace, and the cost (and availability) of land, labor, raw materials, and capital goods can be assumed to vary.
Competitor	Other organizations in the same industry or type of business that provide a good or service to the same set of customers is referred to as a competitor.
Cash flow	In finance, cash flow refers to the amounts of cash being received and spent by a business during a defined period of time, sometimes tied to a specific project. Most of the time they are being used to determine gaps in the liquid position of a company.
Bond	Bond refers to a debt instrument, issued by a borrower and promising a specified stream of payments to the purchaser, usually regular interest payments plus a final repayment of principal.
Double taxation	The taxation of both corporate net income and the dividends paid from this net income when they become the personal income of households a double taxation.
Property	Assets defined in the broadest legal sense. Property includes the unrealized receivables of a cash basis taxpayer, but not services rendered.
Interest payment	The payment to holders of bonds payable, calculated by multiplying the stated rate on the face of the bond by the par, or face, value of the bond. If bonds are issued at a discount or premium, the interest payment does not equal the interest expense.
Exempt	Employees who are not covered by the Fair Labor Standards Act are exempt. Exempt employees are not eligible for overtime pay.
Interest rate	The rate of return on bonds, loans, or deposits. When one speaks of 'the' interest rate, it is usually in a model where there is only one.
Users	Users refer to people in the organization who actually use the product or service purchased by the buying center.
Health insurance	Health insurance is a type of insurance whereby the insurer pays the medical costs of the insured if the insured becomes sick due to covered causes, or due to accidents. The insurer may be a private organization or a government agency.
American Hospital Association	Founded in 1898, the American Hospital Association, located in Chicago, Illinois, is the national organization that represents and serves all types of hospitals, health care networks, and their patients and communities. It provides education for health care leaders and is a source of information on health care issues and trends.
Enabling legislation	The statute by which a legislative body creates an administrative agency is referred to as an enabling legislation.
Capital requirement	The capital requirement is a bank regulation, which sets a framework on how banks and depository institutions must handle their capital. The categorization of assets and capital is highly standardized so that it can be risk weighted.

Chapter 2. The Financial Environment

Chapter 2. The Financial Environment

Enabling	Enabling refers to giving workers the education and tools they need to assume their new decision-making powers.
American Medical Association	The American Medical Association is the largest association of medical doctors in the United States. Its purpose is to advance the interests of physicians, to promote public health, to lobby for medical legislation, and to raise money for medical education.
Subsidiary	A company that is controlled by another company or corporation is a subsidiary.
Form of ownership	Distinguishes retail outlets based on whether individuals, corporate chains, or contractual systems own the outlet is called form of ownership.
Fringe benefits	The rewards other than wages that employees receive from their employers and that include pensions, medical and dental insurance, paid vacations, and sick leaves are referred to as fringe benefits.
Fringe benefit	Benefits such as sick-leave pay, vacation pay, pension plans, and health plans that represent additional compenzation to employees beyond base wages is a fringe benefit.
Contract	A contract is a "promise" or an "agreement" that is enforced or recognized by the law. In the civil law, a contract is considered to be part of the general law of obligations.
Argument	The discussion by counsel for the respective parties of their contentions on the law and the facts of the case being tried in order to aid the jury in arriving at a correct and just conclusion is called argument.
Medicare	Medicare refers to federal program that is financed by payroll taxes and provides for compulsory hospital insurance for senior citizens and low-cost voluntary insurance to help older Americans pay physicians' fees.
Social Security	Social security primarily refers to a field of social welfare concerned with social protection, or protection against socially recognized conditions, including poverty, old age, disability, unemployment, families with children and others.
Premium	Premium refers to the fee charged by an insurance company for an insurance policy. The rate of losses must be relatively predictable: In order to set the premium (prices) insurers must be able to estimate them accurately.
Supplemental Security Income	A federally financed and administered program that provides a uniform nationwide minimum income for the aged, blind, or disabled who do not qualify for benefits under the Old Age, Survivors, and Disability Health Insurance or unemployment is a supplemental security income.
Intermediaries	Intermediaries specialize in information either to bring together two parties to a transaction or to buy in order to sell again.
Health maintenance organization	A Health Maintenance Organization is a fixed, prepaid health care plan that provides comprehensive benefits for employees who are required to use a network of participating providers for all health services.
Comprehensive	A comprehensive refers to a layout accurate in size, color, scheme, and other necessary details to show how a final ad will look. For presentation only, never for reproduction.
Organizational structure	Organizational structure is the way in which the interrelated groups of an organization are constructed. From a managerial point of view the main concerns are ensuring effective communication and coordination.
Beneficiary	The person for whose benefit an insurance policy, trust, will, or contract is established is a beneficiary. In the case of a contract, the beneficiary is called a third-party beneficiary.
Gatekeeper	Gatekeeper refers to an individual who has a strategic position in the network that allows

Chapter 2. The Financial Environment

Chapter 2. The Financial Environment

	him or her to control information moving in either direction through a channel.
Preferred provider organization	A group of health care providers who contract with employers, insurance companies, and so forth to provide health care at a reduced fee is called preferred provider organization.
Managerial Accounting	Managerial accounting is the branch of accounting that uses both past and future data in providing information that management uses in conducting daily operations in planning future operations, and in developing overall business strategies.
Trend	Trend refers to the long-term movement of an economic variable, such as its average rate of increase or decrease over enough years to encompass several business cycles.
Bargaining power	Bargaining power refers to the ability to influence the setting of prices or wages, usually arising from some sort of monopoly or monopsony position
Discount	The difference between the face value of a bond and its selling price, when a bond is sold for less than its face value it's referred to as a discount.
Administrative cost	An administrative cost is all executive, organizational, and clerical costs associated with the general management of an organization rather than with manufacturing, marketing, or selling
Financial accounting	Financial accounting is the branch of accountancy concerned with the preparation of financial statements for external decision makers, such as stockholders, suppliers, banks and government agencies. The fundamental need for financial accounting is to reduce principal-agent problem by measuring and monitoring agents' performance.
Home equity loans	Home equity loans refer to loans that utilize the personal residence of the taxpayer as security. The interest on such loans may be deductible as qualified residence interest.
Mortgage	Mortgage refers to a note payable issued for property, such as a house, usually repaid in equal installments consisting of part principle and part interest, over a specified period.
Purchasing	Purchasing refers to the function in a firm that searches for quality material resources, finds the best suppliers, and negotiates the best price for goods and services.
Churning	Churning is the practice of executing trades for an investment account by a salesman or broker in order to generate commissions from the account. It is a breach of securities law in many jurisdictions, and it is generally actionable by the account holder for the return of the commissions paid.
Unbundling	Relying on more than one financial technique to transfer funds across borders is called unbundling.
Financial risk	The risk related to the inability of the firm to meet its debt obligations as they come due is called financial risk.
Utilization review	Utilization review is a technique used by some insurers and employers to evaluate health care on the basis of appropriateness, necessity, and quality.
Closing	The finalization of a real estate sales transaction that passes title to the property from the seller to the buyer is referred to as a closing. Closing is a sales term which refers to the process of making a sale. It refers to reaching the final step, which may be an exchange of money or acquiring a signature.
Contribution	In business organization law, the cash or property contributed to a business by its owners is referred to as contribution.
Conflict of interest	A conflict that occurs when a corporate officer or director enters into a transaction with the corporation in which he or she has a personal interest is a conflict of interest.

Go to **Cram101.com** for the Practice Tests for this Chapter.

Chapter 2. The Financial Environment

Chapter 2. The Financial Environment

Health maintenance organizations	Health care providers that contract with employers, insurance companies, labor unions, or government units to provide health care for their workers or others who are insured are referred to as health maintenance organizations.
Net income	Net income is equal to the income that a firm has after subtracting costs and expenses from the total revenue. Expenses will typically include tax expense.
Broker	In commerce, a broker is a party that mediates between a buyer and a seller. A broker who also acts as a seller or as a buyer becomes a principal party to the deal.
Financial market	In economics, a financial market is a mechanism which allows people to trade money for securities or commodities such as gold or other precious metals. In general, any commodity market might be considered to be a financial market, if the usual purpose of traders is not the immediate consumption of the commodity, but rather as a means of delaying or accelerating consumption over time.
Developed country	A developed country is one that enjoys a relatively high standard of living derived through an industrialized, diversified economy. Countries with a very high Human Development Index are generally considered developed countries.
Equity capital	Equity capital refers to money raized from within the firm or through the sale of ownership in the firm.
Customer service	The ability of logistics management to satisfy users in terms of time, dependability, communication, and convenience is called the customer service.
Audit	An examination of the financial reports to ensure that they represent what they claim and conform with generally accepted accounting principles is referred to as audit.
Administration	Administration refers to the management and direction of the affairs of governments and institutions; a collective term for all policymaking officials of a government; the execution and implementation of public policy.
Harvard Business Review	Harvard Business Review is a research-based magazine written for business practitioners, it claims a high ranking business readership and enjoys the reverence of academics, executives, and management consultants. It has been the frequent publishing home for well known scholars and management thinkers.
Agency cost	An agency cost is the cost incurred by an organization that is associated with problems such as divergent management-shareholder objectives and information asymmetry.
Journal	Book of original entry, in which transactions are recorded in a general ledger system, is referred to as a journal.
Financial perspective	Financial perspective is one of the four standard perspectives used with the Balanced Scorecard. Financial perspective measures inform an organization whether strategy execution, which is detailed through measures in the other three perspectives, is leading to improved bottom line results.

Chapter 2. The Financial Environment

Chapter 3. Financial Accounting Basics and the Income Statement

Financial accounting	Financial accounting is the branch of accountancy concerned with the preparation of financial statements for external decision makers, such as stockholders, suppliers, banks and government agencies. The fundamental need for financial accounting is to reduce principal-agent problem by measuring and monitoring agents' performance.
Accounting	A system that collects and processes financial information about an organization and reports that information to decision makers is referred to as accounting.
Income statement	Income statement refers to a financial statement that presents the revenues and expenses and resulting net income or net loss of a company for a specific period of time.
Net income	Net income is equal to the income that a firm has after subtracting costs and expenses from the total revenue. Expenses will typically include tax expense.
Expense	In accounting, an expense represents an event in which an asset is used up or a liability is incurred. In terms of the accounting equation, expenses reduce owners' equity.
Cash flow	In finance, cash flow refers to the amounts of cash being received and spent by a business during a defined period of time, sometimes tied to a specific project. Most of the time they are being used to determine gaps in the liquid position of a company.
Liability	A liability is a present obligation of the enterprise arizing from past events, the settlement of which is expected to result in an outflow from the enterprise of resources embodying economic benefits.
Equity	Equity is the name given to the set of legal principles, in countries following the English common law tradition, which supplement strict rules of law where their application would operate harshly, so as to achieve what is sometimes referred to as "natural justice."
Asset	An item of property, such as land, capital, money, a share in ownership, or a claim on others for future payment, such as a bond or a bank deposit is an asset.
Financial statement	Financial statement refers to a summary of all the transactions that have occurred over a particular period.
Physical asset	A physical asset is an item of economic value that has a tangible or material existence. A physical asset usually refers to cash, equipment, inventory and properties owned by a business.
Foundation	A Foundation is a type of philanthropic organization set up by either individuals or institutions as a legal entity (either as a corporation or trust) with the purpose of distributing grants to support causes in line with the goals of the foundation.
Production	The creation of finished goods and services using the factors of production: land, labor, capital, entrepreneurship, and knowledge.
Operation	A standardized method or technique that is performed repetitively, often on different materials resulting in different finished goods is called an operation.
Merchant	Under the Uniform Commercial Code, one who regularly deals in goods of the kind sold in the contract at issue, or holds himself out as having special knowledge or skill relevant to such goods, or who makes the sale through an agent who regularly deals in such goods or claims such knowledge or skill is referred to as merchant.
Economy	The income, expenditures, and resources that affect the cost of running a business and household are called an economy.
Profit	Profit refers to the return to the resource entrepreneurial ability; total revenue minus total cost.
Lender	Suppliers and financial institutions that lend money to companies is referred to as a lender.

Chapter 3. Financial Accounting Basics and the Income Statement

Chapter 3. Financial Accounting Basics and the Income Statement

Economic system	Economic system refers to a particular set of institutional arrangements and a coordinating mechanism for solving the economizing problem; a method of organizing an economy, of which the market system and the command system are the two general types.
Historical cost	In accounting terminology, historical cost describes the original cost of an asset at the time of purchase or payment as opposed to its market value
Balance sheet	A statement of the assets, liabilities, and net worth of a firm or individual at some given time often at the end of its "fiscal year," is referred to as a balance sheet.
Balance	In banking and accountancy, the outstanding balance is the amount of money owned, (or due), that remains in a deposit account (or a loan account) at a given date, after all past remittances, payments and withdrawal have been accounted for. It can be positive (then, in the balance sheet of a firm, it is an asset) or negative (a liability).
Interest	In finance and economics, interest is the price paid by a borrower for the use of a lender's money. In other words, interest is the amount of paid to "rent" money for a period of time.
Users	Users refer to people in the organization who actually use the product or service purchased by the buying center.
Stakeholder	A stakeholder is an individual or group with a vested interest in or expectation for organizational performance. Usually stakeholders can either have an effect on or are affected by an organization.
Creditor	A person to whom a debt or legal obligation is owed, and who has the right to enforce payment of that debt or obligation is referred to as creditor.
Service	Service refers to a "non tangible product" that is not embodied in a physical good and that typically effects some change in another product, person, or institution. Contrasts with good.
Capital	Capital generally refers to financial wealth, especially that used to start or maintain a business. In classical economics, capital is one of four factors of production, the others being land and labor and entrepreneurship.
Supply	Supply is the aggregate amount of any material good that can be called into being at a certain price point; it comprises one half of the equation of supply and demand. In classical economic theory, a curve representing supply is one of the factors that produce price.
Fund	Independent accounting entity with a self-balancing set of accounts segregated for the purposes of carrying on specific activities is referred to as a fund.
Equity capital	Equity capital refers to money raized from within the firm or through the sale of ownership in the firm.
Debt capital	Debt capital refers to funds raized through various forms of borrowing to finance a company that must be repaid.
Stockholder	A stockholder is an individual or company (including a corporation) that legally owns one or more shares of stock in a joined stock company. The shareholders are the owners of a corporation. Companies listed at the stock market strive to enhance shareholder value.
Bankruptcy	Bankruptcy is a legally declared inability or impairment of ability of an individual or organization to pay their creditors.
Federal government	Federal government refers to the government of the United States, as distinct from the state and local governments.
Great Depression	The period of severe economic contraction and high unemployment that began in 1929 and continued throughout the 1930s is referred to as the Great Depression.

Go to **Cram101.com** for the Practice Tests for this Chapter.

Chapter 3. Financial Accounting Basics and the Income Statement

Chapter 3. Financial Accounting Basics and the Income Statement

Disclosure	Disclosure means the giving out of information, either voluntarily or to be in compliance with legal regulations or workplace rules.
Depression	Depression refers to a prolonged period characterized by high unemployment, low output and investment, depressed business confidence, falling prices, and widespread business failures. A milder form of business downturn is a recession.
Regulation	Regulation refers to restrictions state and federal laws place on business with regard to the conduct of its activities.
Industry	A group of firms that produce identical or similar products is an industry. It is also used specifically to refer to an area of economic production focused on manufacturing which involves large amounts of capital investment before any profit can be realized, also called "heavy industry".
Security	Security refers to a claim on the borrower future income that is sold by the borrower to the lender. A security is a type of transferable interest representing financial value.
Securities and exchange commission	Securities and exchange commission refers to U.S. government agency that determines the financial statements that public companies must provide to stockholders and the measurement rules that they must use in producing those statements.
Regulatory agency	Regulatory agency refers to an agency, commission, or board established by the Federal government or a state government to regulates businesses in the public interest.
Authority	Authority in agency law, refers to an agent's ability to affect his principal's legal relations with third parties. Also used to refer to an actor's legal power or ability to do something. In addition, sometimes used to refer to a statute, case, or other legal source that justifies a particular result.
Exchange	The trade of things of value between buyer and seller so that each is better off after the trade is called the exchange.
Gain	In finance, gain is a profit or an increase in value of an investment such as a stock or bond. Gain is calculated by fair market value or the proceeds from the sale of the investment minus the sum of the purchase price and all costs associated with it.
American Institute of Certified Public Accountants	With over 350,000 CPA members (in 2005), the American Institute of Certified Public Accountants is the largest CPA professional organization in the United States of America. Approximately 40% of its members are engaged in the practice of public accounting, in areas such as auditing, accounting, taxation, general business consulting, business valuation, personal financial planning and business technology.
Certified Public Accountant	Certified Public Accountant refers to an individual in the United States who have passed the Uniform Certified Public Accountant Examination and have met additional state education and experience requirements for certification as a Certified Public Accountant.
Committee	A long-lasting, sometimes permanent team in the organization structure created to deal with tasks that recur regularly is the committee.
Preparation	Preparation refers to usually the first stage in the creative process. It includes education and formal training.
External audit	The main difference between Internal and External auditing is that External audit focusses on financial statements, whereas Internal Audit focusses on processes, be it financial or not.
Audit	An examination of the financial reports to ensure that they represent what they claim and conform with generally accepted accounting principles is referred to as audit.
Qualified opinion	A qualified opinion is one issued by a CPA that means that for the most part, the company's financial statements are in compliance with GAAP, but the auditors have reservations about

Chapter 3. Financial Accounting Basics and the Income Statement

Chapter 3. Financial Accounting Basics and the Income Statement

	something in the statements or have other reasons not to give a fully unqualified opinion; reasons that a qualified opinion is being issued are explained in the auditor's report.
Adverse opinion	The adverse opinion is an audit opinion for a set of financial statements issued by a certified public accountant that means that part of or all of the financial statements are not in compliance with GAAP and the auditors believe this noncompliance would be material to the average prudent investor.
Internal auditor	An accountant employed within a firm who reviews the accounting procedures, records, and reports in both the controller's and treasurer's areas of responsibility is referred to as an internal auditor.
Management	Management characterizes the process of leading and directing all or part of an organization, often a business, through the deployment and manipulation of resources. Early twentieth-century management writer Mary Parker Follett defined management as "the art of getting things done through people."
Firm	An organization that employs resources to produce a good or service for profit and owns and operates one or more plants is referred to as a firm.
Audit committee	Audit committee in corporation law, a committee of the board that recommends and supervises the public accountant who audits the corporation's financial records.
Board of directors	The group of individuals elected by the stockholders of a corporation to oversee its operations is a board of directors.
Chief executive officer	A chief executive officer is the highest-ranking corporate officer or executive officer of a corporation, or agency. In closely held corporations, it is general business culture that the office chief executive officer is also the chairman of the board.
Chief financial officer	Chief financial officer refers to executive responsible for overseeing the financial operations of an organization.
Negotiation	Negotiation is the process whereby interested parties resolve disputes, agree upon courses of action, bargain for individual or collective advantage, and/or attempt to craft outcomes which serve their mutual interests.
Compromise	Compromise occurs when the interaction is moderately important to meeting goals and the goals are neither completely compatible nor completely incompatible.
Going concern	A going concern describes a business that functions without the intention or threat of liquidation for the foreseeable future. Accountants and auditors may be required to evaluate and disclose whether a company is no longer a going concern, or is at risk of ceasing to be
Purchasing power	The amount of goods that money will buy, usually measured by the CPI is referred to as purchasing power.
Purchasing	Purchasing refers to the function in a firm that searches for quality material resources, finds the best suppliers, and negotiates the best price for goods and services.
Materiality	Materiality refers to the constraint of determining whether an item is large enough to likely influence the decision of an investor or creditor.
Core business	The core business of an organization is an idealized construct intended to express that organization's "main" or "essential" activity.
Inventory	Tangible property held for sale in the normal course of business or used in producing goods or services for sale is an inventory.
Core	A core is the set of feasible allocations in an economy that cannot be improved upon by subset of the set of the economy's consumers (a coalition). In construction, when the force

Chapter 3. Financial Accounting Basics and the Income Statement

Chapter 3. Financial Accounting Basics and the Income Statement

	in an element is within a certain center section, the core, the element will only be under compression.
Comparability	Ability to compare the accounting information of different companies because they use the same accounting principles is known as comparability.
Annual financial statement	Annual financial statement refers to a statement provided to the shareholders that contains a balance sheet, an income statement, and a statement of changes in shareholder equity.
Accrual accounting	Method of accounting that records the effects of accounting events in the period in which such events occur regardless of when cash is exchanged is accrual accounting.
Accrual method	Accrual method refers to a method of accounting that reflects expenses incurred and income earned during the period of the transaction, instead of when cash changes hands.
Accrual	An accrual is an accounting event in which the transaction is recognized when the action takes place, instead of when cash is disbursed or received.
Cash Accounting	a method of bookkeeping in which income is considered earned when received and expenses are not taken into account until paid is cash accounting. Similarly, cash accounting does not generally recognise non-cash expenses such as depreciation.
Accrual basis accounting	Accounting basis in which transactions that change a company's financial statements are recorded in the periods in which the events occur, rather than in the periods in which the company receives or pays cash are referred to as accrual basis accounting.
Financial transaction	A financial transaction involves a change in the status of the finances of two or more businesses or individuals.
Accrual basis	Accrual basis refers to recording revenues when earned and expenses when incurred, regardless of the timing of cash receipts or payments.
Revenue	Revenue is a U.S. business term for the amount of money that a company receives from its activities, mostly from sales of products and/or services to customers.
Conversion	Conversion refers to any distinct act of dominion wrongfully exerted over another's personal property in denial of or inconsistent with his rights therein. That tort committed by a person who deals with chattels not belonging to him in a manner that is inconsistent with the ownership of the lawful owner.
Cash basis	Cash basis is a bookkeeping method that recognizes revenue and expenses at the time of cash receipt or payment. It is the opposite of Accrual Basis.
Matching principle	The matching principle indictates that when it is reasonable to do so, expenses should be matched with revenues. When expenses are matched with revenues, they are not recognized until the associated revenue is also recognized.
Matching	Matching refers to an accounting concept that establishes when expenses are recognized. Expenses are matched with the revenues they helped to generate and are recognized when those revenues are recognized.
Preference	The act of a debtor in paying or securing one or more of his creditors in a manner more favorable to them than to other creditors or to the exclusion of such other creditors is a preference. In the absence of statute, a preference is perfectly good, but to be legal it must be bona fide, and not a mere subterfuge of the debtor to secure a future benefit to himself or to prevent the application of his property to his debts.
Enterprise	Enterprise refers to another name for a business organization. Other similar terms are business firm, sometimes simply business, sometimes simply firm, as well as company, and entity.

Chapter 3. Financial Accounting Basics and the Income Statement

Chapter 3. Financial Accounting Basics and the Income Statement

General ledger	General ledger refers to a ledger that contains all asset, liability, and stockholders' equity accounts. The general ledger is a summary of all of the transactions that occur in the company. It is taken directly from the general journal, where each transaction is recorded.
Subsidiary	A company that is controlled by another company or corporation is a subsidiary.
Ledger	Ledger refers to a specialized accounting book in which information from accounting journals is accumulated into specific categories and posted so that managers can find all the information about one account in the same place.
Chart of accounts	A chart of accounts is a list of all accounts tracked by a single accounting system, and should be designed to capture financial information to make good financial decisions.
Permanent accounts	The balance sheet accounts that carry their ending balances into the next accounting period are called permanent accounts.
Interest payment	The payment to holders of bonds payable, calculated by multiplying the stated rate on the face of the bond by the par, or face, value of the bond. If bonds are issued at a discount or premium, the interest payment does not equal the interest expense.
Temporary accounts	Revenue, expense, and dividend accounts whose balances are transferred to Retained Earnings at the end of an accounting period are called temporary accounts.
Contra account	Contra account refers to an account that normally has a balance opposite to that of the other accounts in a particular category. An account whose balance is subtracted from an associated account in the financial statement.
Depreciation expense	Depreciation expense refers to the amount recognized as an expense in one period resulting from the periodic recognition of the used portion of the cost of a long-term tangible asset over its life.
Depreciation	Depreciation is an accounting and finance term for the method of attributing the cost of an asset across the useful life of the asset. Depreciation is a reduction in the value of a currency in floating exchange rate.
Journal	Book of original entry, in which transactions are recorded in a general ledger system, is referred to as a journal.
Debit	Debit refers to recording as negative in the balance of payments, any transaction that gives rise to a payment out of the country, such as an import, the purchase of an asset, or lending to foreigners. Opposite of credit.
Credit	Credit refers to a recording as positive in the balance of payments, any transaction that gives rise to a payment into the country, such as an export, the sale of an asset, or borrowing from abroad.
Statement of cash flow	Reports inflows and outflows of cash during the accounting period in the categories of operating, investing, and financing is a statement of cash flow.
Annual report	An annual report is prepared by corporate management that presents financial information including financial statements, footnotes, and the management discussion and analysis.
Insurance	Insurance refers to a system by which individuals can reduce their exposure to risk of large losses by spreading the risks among a large number of persons.
Interest expense	The cost a business incurs to borrow money. With respect to bonds payable, the interest expense is calculated by multiplying the market rate of interest by the carrying value of the bonds on the date of the payment.
Lease	A contract for the possession and use of land or other property, including goods, on one side, and a recompense of rent or other income on the other is the lease.

Go to **Cram101.com** for the Practice Tests for this Chapter.

Chapter 3. Financial Accounting Basics and the Income Statement

Chapter 3. Financial Accounting Basics and the Income Statement

Net loss	Net loss refers to the amount by which expenses exceed revenues. The difference between income received and expenses, when expenses are greater.
Bad debt	In accounting and finance, bad debt is the portion of receivables that can no longer be collected, typically from accounts receivable or loans. Bad debt in accounting is considered an expense.
Discount	The difference between the face value of a bond and its selling price, when a bond is sold for less than its face value it's referred to as a discount.
Policy	Similar to a script in that a policy can be a less than completely rational decision-making method. Involves the use of a pre-existing set of decision steps for any problem that presents itself.
Final settlement	Final settlement occurs when the payor bank pays the check in cash, settles for the check without having a right to revoke the settlement, or fails to dishonor the check within certain statutory time periods.
Ancillary	An ancillary receiver is a receiver who has been appointed in aid of, and in subordination to, the primary receiver.
Premium	Premium refers to the fee charged by an insurance company for an insurance policy. The rate of losses must be relatively predictable: In order to set the premium (prices) insurers must be able to estimate them accurately.
Contract	A contract is a "promise" or an "agreement" that is enforced or recognized by the law. In the civil law, a contract is considered to be part of the general law of obligations.
Investment	Investment refers to spending for the production and accumulation of capital and additions to inventories. In a financial sense, buying an asset with the expectation of making a return.
Interest income	Interest income refers to payments of income to those who supply the economy with capital.
Contribution	In business organization law, the cash or property contributed to a business by its owners is referred to as contribution.
Charitable contributions	Charitable contributions refers to contributions that are tax deductible if made to qualified nonprofit charitable organizations. A cash basis taxpayer is entitled to a deduction solely in the year of payment.
Allowance	Reduction in the selling price of goods extended to the buyer because the goods are defective or of lower quality than the buyer ordered and to encourage a buyer to keep merchandise that would otherwise be returned is the allowance.
Complexity	The technical sophistication of the product and hence the amount of understanding required to use it is referred to as complexity. It is the opposite of simplicity.
Cost structure	The relative proportion of an organization's fixed, variable, and mixed costs is referred to as cost structure.
Labor	People's physical and mental talents and efforts that are used to help produce goods and services are called labor.
Accounting information system	The system of collecting and processing transaction data and communicating financial information to interested parties is called the accounting information system.
Information system	An information system is a system whether automated or manual, that comprises people, machines, and/or methods organized to collect, process, transmit, and disseminate data that represent user information.
Managerial	Managerial accounting is the branch of accounting that uses both past and future data in

Chapter 3. Financial Accounting Basics and the Income Statement

Chapter 3. Financial Accounting Basics and the Income Statement

Accounting	providing information that management uses in conducting daily operations in planning future operations, and in developing overall business strategies.
Stock	In financial terminology, stock is the capital raized by a corporation, through the issuance and sale of shares.
Malfeasance	Malfeasance refers to the doing of an act that a person ought not to do at all. It is to be distinguished from misfeasance; the improper doing of an act that a person might lawfully do.
Property	Assets defined in the broadest legal sense. Property includes the unrealized receivables of a cash basis taxpayer, but not services rendered.
Fixed asset	Fixed asset, also known as property, plant, and equipment (PP&E), is a term used in accountancy for assets and property which cannot easily be converted into cash. This can be compared with current assets such as cash or bank accounts, which are described as liquid assets. In most cases, only tangible assets are referred to as fixed.
Acquisition cost	Net cash equivalent amount paid or to be paid for the asset is an acquisition cost. e expense undertaken to acquire new business. The concept applies to both agents and companies. The largest portion of an insurer's acquisition cost is agent's or sales representative's commission or bonus.
Acquisition	A company's purchase of the property and obligations of another company is an acquisition.
Allocate	Allocate refers to the assignment of income for various tax purposes. A multistate corporation's nonbusiness income usually is distributed to the state where the nonbusiness assets are located; it is not apportioned with the rest of the entity's income.
Market value	Market value refers to the price of an asset agreed on between a willing buyer and a willing seller; the price an asset could demand if it is sold on the open market.
Market	A market is, as defined in economics, a social arrangement that allows buyers and sellers to discover information and carry out a voluntary exchange of goods or services.
Salvage value	In accounting, the salvage value of an asset is its remaining value after depreciation. The estimated value of an asset at the end of its useful life.
Useful life	The length of service of a productive facility or piece of equipment is its useful life. The period of time during which an asset will have economic value and be usable.
Capital structure	Capital Structure refers to the way a corporation finances itself through some combination of equity sales, equity options, bonds, and loans. Optimal capital structure refers to the particular combination that minimizes the cost of capital while maximizing the stock price.
Closing	The finalization of a real estate sales transaction that passes title to the property from the seller to the buyer is referred to as a closing. Closing is a sales term which refers to the process of making a sale. It refers to reaching the final step, which may be an exchange of money or acquiring a signature.
Bottom line	The bottom line is net income on the last line of a income statement.
Net assets	Net assets refers to portion of the assets remaining after the creditors' claims have been satisfied; also called equity or residual interest.
Dividend	Amount of corporate profits paid out for each share of stock is referred to as dividend.
Economic income	The amount of money a household can spend during a given period without increasing or decreasing its net assets. Wages, salaries, dividends, interest income, transfer payments, rents, and so forth are sources of economic income.
Operating expense	In throughput accounting, the cost accounting aspect of Theory of Constraints (TOC), operating expense is the money spent turning inventory into throughput. In TOC, operating

Chapter 3. Financial Accounting Basics and the Income Statement

Chapter 3. Financial Accounting Basics and the Income Statement

	expense is limited to costs that vary strictly with the quantity produced, like raw materials and purchased components.
Accumulated depreciation	Accumulated depreciation refers to the total depreciation that has been reported as depreciation expense for the entire life of a long-term tangible asset. It is a contra-asset account.
Cash value	The cash value of an insurance policy is the amount available to the policy holder in cash upon cancellation of the policy. This term is normally used with a whole life policy in which a portion of the premiums go toward an investment. The cash value is the value of this investment at any particular time.
Form of ownership	Distinguishes retail outlets based on whether individuals, corporate chains, or contractual systems own the outlet is called form of ownership.
Ratio analysis	Ratio analysis refers to an analytical tool designed to identify significant relationships; measures the proportional relationship between two financial statement amounts.
Profit margin	Profit margin is a measure of profitability. It is calculated using a formula and written as a percentage or a number. Profit margin = Net income before tax and interest / Revenue.
Total revenue	Total revenue refers to the total number of dollars received by a firm from the sale of a product; equal to the total expenditures for the product produced by the firm; equal to the quantity sold multiplied by the price at which it is sold.
Margin	A deposit by a buyer in stocks with a seller or a stockbroker, as security to cover fluctuations in the market in reference to stocks that the buyer has purchased but for which he has not paid is a margin. Commodities are also traded on margin.
Trend	Trend refers to the long-term movement of an economic variable, such as its average rate of increase or decrease over enough years to encompass several business cycles.
Brief	Brief refers to a statement of a party's case or legal arguments, usually prepared by an attorney. Also used to make legal arguments before appellate courts.
Generally accepted accounting principles	Generally accepted accounting principles refers to the standard framework of guidelines for financial accounting. It includes the standards, conventions, and rules accountants follow in recording and summarizing transactions, and in the preparation of financial statements.
Economic cost	Economic cost refers to payments made or incomes forgone to obtain and retain the services of a resource.
Corporation	A legal entity chartered by a state or the Federal government that is distinct and separate from the individuals who own it is a corporation. This separation gives the corporation unique powers which other legal entities lack.
Accounting Standards Board	The role of the Accounting Standards Board is to issue accounting standards in the United Kingdom. It is recognized for that purpose under the Companies Act 1985. It took over the task of setting accounting standards from the Accounting Standards Committee (ASC) in 1990.
Financial instrument	Formal or legal documents in writing, such as contracts, deeds, wills, bonds, leases, and mortgages is referred to as a financial instrument.
Instrument	Instrument refers to an economic variable that is controlled by policy makers and can be used to influence other variables, called targets. Examples are monetary and fiscal policies used to achieve external and internal balance.
Option	A contract that gives the purchaser the option to buy or sell the underlying financial instrument at a specified price, called the exercise price or strike price, within a specific period of time.

Chapter 3. Financial Accounting Basics and the Income Statement

Chapter 3. Financial Accounting Basics and the Income Statement

Financial management	The job of managing a firm's resources so it can meet its goals and objectives is called financial management.
Administration	Administration refers to the management and direction of the affairs of governments and institutions; a collective term for all policymaking officials of a government; the execution and implementation of public policy.

Chapter 3. Financial Accounting Basics and the Income Statement

Chapter 4. The Balance Sheet and Statement of Cash Flows

Income statement	Income statement refers to a financial statement that presents the revenues and expenses and resulting net income or net loss of a company for a specific period of time.
Balance sheet	A statement of the assets, liabilities, and net worth of a firm or individual at some given time often at the end of its "fiscal year," is referred to as a balance sheet.
Balance	In banking and accountancy, the outstanding balance is the amount of money owned, (or due), that remains in a deposit account (or a loan account) at a given date, after all past remittances, payments and withdrawal have been accounted for. It can be positive (then, in the balance sheet of a firm, it is an asset) or negative (a liability).
Cash flow	In finance, cash flow refers to the amounts of cash being received and spent by a business during a defined period of time, sometimes tied to a specific project. Most of the time they are being used to determine gaps in the liquid position of a company.
Statement of cash flow	Reports inflows and outflows of cash during the accounting period in the categories of operating, investing, and financing is a statement of cash flow.
Operation	A standardized method or technique that is performed repetitively, often on different materials resulting in different finished goods is called an operation.
Revenue	Revenue is a U.S. business term for the amount of money that a company receives from its activities, mostly from sales of products and/or services to customers.
Financial statement	Financial statement refers to a summary of all the transactions that have occurred over a particular period.
Asset	An item of property, such as land, capital, money, a share in ownership, or a claim on others for future payment, such as a bond or a bank deposit is an asset.
Net income	Net income is equal to the income that a firm has after subtracting costs and expenses from the total revenue. Expenses will typically include tax expense.
Composition	An out-of-court settlement in which creditors agree to accept a fractional settlement on their original claim is referred to as composition.
Accounting	A system that collects and processes financial information about an organization and reports that information to decision makers is referred to as accounting.
Liability	A liability is a present obligation of the enterprise arizing from past events, the settlement of which is expected to result in an outflow from the enterprise of resources embodying economic benefits.
Equity	Equity is the name given to the set of legal principles, in countries following the English common law tradition, which supplement strict rules of law where their application would operate harshly, so as to achieve what is sometimes referred to as "natural justice."
Capital	Capital generally refers to financial wealth, especially that used to start or maintain a business. In classical economics, capital is one of four factors of production, the others being land and labor and entrepreneurship.
Residual	Residual payments can refer to an ongoing stream of payments in respect of the completion of past achievements.
Contract	A contract is a "promise" or an "agreement" that is enforced or recognized by the law. In the civil law, a contract is considered to be part of the general law of obligations.
Basic accounting equation	Assets(A) = liabilities(L) + stockholders' equity(E) is called the basic accounting equation.
Accounting	Expression of the relationship between the assets and the claims on those assets is referred

Chapter 4. The Balance Sheet and Statement of Cash Flows

Chapter 4. The Balance Sheet and Statement of Cash Flows

equation	to as the accounting equation, specifically Assets = Liabilities + Owners' equity.
Liquidated	Damages made certain by the prior agreement of the parties are called liquidated.
Creditor	A person to whom a debt or legal obligation is owed, and who has the right to enforce payment of that debt or obligation is referred to as creditor.
Service	Service refers to a "non tangible product" that is not embodied in a physical good and that typically effects some change in another product, person, or institution. Contrasts with good.
Closing date	Date when all advertising material must be submitted to a publication is referred to as the closing date.
Closing	The finalization of a real estate sales transaction that passes title to the property from the seller to the buyer is referred to as a closing. Closing is a sales term which refers to the process of making a sale. It refers to reaching the final step, which may be an exchange of money or acquiring a signature.
Current asset	A current asset is an asset on the balance sheet which is expected to be sold or otherwise used up in the near future, usually within one year.
Current liability	Current liability refers to a debt that can reasonably be expected to be paid from existing current assets or through the creation of other current liabilities, within one year or the operating cycle, whichever is longer.
Conversion	Conversion refers to any distinct act of dominion wrongfully exerted over another's personal property in denial of or inconsistent with his rights therein. That tort committed by a person who deals with chattels not belonging to him in a manner that is inconsistent with the ownership of the lawful owner.
Liquidity	Liquidity refers to the capacity to turn assets into cash, or the amount of assets in a portfolio that have that capacity.
Fund	Independent accounting entity with a self-balancing set of accounts segregated for the purposes of carrying on specific activities is referred to as a fund.
Commercial paper	Commercial paper is a money market security issued by large banks and corporations. It is generally not used to finance long-term investments but rather for purchases of inventory or to manage working capital. It is commonly bought by money funds (the issuing amounts are often too high for individual investors), and is generally regarded as a very safe investment.
Demand deposit	Demand deposit refers to a bank deposit that can be withdrawn 'on demand.' The term usually refers only to checking accounts, even though depositors in many other kinds of accounts may be able to write checks and regard their deposits as readily available.
Treasury bills	Short-term obligations of the federal government are treasury bills. They are like zero coupon bonds in that they do not pay interest prior to maturity; instead they are sold at a discount of the par value to create a positive yield to maturity.
Money market	The money market, in macroeconomics and international finance, refers to the equilibration of demand for a country's domestic money to its money supply; market for short-term financial instruments.
Mutual fund	A mutual fund is a form of collective investment that pools money from many investors and invests the money in stocks, bonds, short-term money market instruments, and/or other securities. In a mutual fund, the fund manager trades the fund's underlying securities, realizing capital gains or loss, and collects the dividend or interest income.
Investment	Investment refers to spending for the production and accumulation of capital and additions to

Chapter 4. The Balance Sheet and Statement of Cash Flows

Chapter 4. The Balance Sheet and Statement of Cash Flows

	inventories. In a financial sense, buying an asset with the expectation of making a return.
Security	Security refers to a claim on the borrower future income that is sold by the borrower to the lender. A security is a type of transferable interest representing financial value.
Market	A market is, as defined in economics, a social arrangement that allows buyers and sellers to discover information and carry out a voluntary exchange of goods or services.
Money market mutual fund	Money market mutual fund refers to a fund operated by a financial institution that sells shares in the fund and holds liquid assets such as U.S. Treasury bills and short-term commercial bills.
Marketable securities	Marketable securities refer to securities that are readily traded in the secondary securities market.
Interest	In finance and economics, interest is the price paid by a borrower for the use of a lender's money. In other words, interest is the amount of paid to "rent" money for a period of time.
Holding	The holding is a court's determination of a matter of law based on the issue presented in the particular case. In other words: under this law, with these facts, this result.
Accounts receivable	Accounts receivable is one of a series of accounting transactions dealing with the billing of customers which owe money to a person, company or organization for goods and services that have been provided to the customer. This is typically done in a one person organization by writing an invoice and mailing or delivering it to each customer.
Allowance	Reduction in the selling price of goods extended to the buyer because the goods are defective or of lower quality than the buyer ordered and to encourage a buyer to keep merchandise that would otherwise be returned is the allowance.
Bad debt	In accounting and finance, bad debt is the portion of receivables that can no longer be collected, typically from accounts receivable or loans. Bad debt in accounting is considered an expense.
Discount	The difference between the face value of a bond and its selling price, when a bond is sold for less than its face value it's referred to as a discount.
Managerial Accounting	Managerial accounting is the branch of accounting that uses both past and future data in providing information that management uses in conducting daily operations in planning future operations, and in developing overall business strategies.
Operating expense	In throughput accounting, the cost accounting aspect of Theory of Constraints (TOC), operating expense is the money spent turning inventory into throughput. In TOC, operating expense is limited to costs that vary strictly with the quantity produced, like raw materials and purchased components.
Expense	In accounting, an expense represents an event in which an asset is used up or a liability is incurred. In terms of the accounting equation, expenses reduce owners' equity.
Inventory	Tangible property held for sale in the normal course of business or used in producing goods or services for sale is an inventory.
Supply	Supply is the aggregate amount of any material good that can be called into being at a certain price point; it comprises one half of the equation of supply and demand. In classical economic theory, a curve representing supply is one of the factors that produce price.
Safety stock	Safety stock is additional inventory planned to buffer against the variability in supply and demand plans, that could otherwise result in inventory shortages.
Stock	In financial terminology, stock is the capital raized by a corporation, through the issuance and sale of shares.

Go to **Cram101.com** for the Practice Tests for this Chapter.

Chapter 4. The Balance Sheet and Statement of Cash Flows

Chapter 4. The Balance Sheet and Statement of Cash Flows

Interest income	Interest income refers to payments of income to those who supply the economy with capital.
Asset management	Asset management is the method that a company uses to track fixed assets, for example factory equipment, desks and chairs, computers, even buildings. Although the exact details of the task varies widely from company to company, asset management often includes tracking the physical location of assets, managing demand for scarce resources, and accounting tasks such as amortization.
Management	Management characterizes the process of leading and directing all or part of an organization, often a business, through the deployment and manipulation of resources. Early twentieth-century management writer Mary Parker Follett defined management as "the art of getting things done through people."
Maturity	Maturity refers to the final payment date of a loan or other financial instrument, after which point no further interest or principal need be paid.
Fair market value	Fair market value refers to the amount at which property would change hands between a willing buyer and a willing seller, neither being under any compulsion to buy or to sell, and both having reasonable knowledge of the relevant facts.
Market value	Market value refers to the price of an asset agreed on between a willing buyer and a willing seller; the price an asset could demand if it is sold on the open market.
Gain	In finance, gain is a profit or an increase in value of an investment such as a stock or bond. Gain is calculated by fair market value or the proceeds from the sale of the investment minus the sum of the purchase price and all costs associated with it.
Working capital	The dollar difference between total current assets and total current liabilities is called working capital.
Carrying costs	Carrying costs refers to costs that arise while holding an inventory of goods for sale.
Carrying cost	The cost to hold an asset, usually inventory is called a carrying cost. For inventory, a carrying cost includes such items as interest, warehousing costs, insurance, and material-handling expenses.
Dividend	Amount of corporate profits paid out for each share of stock is referred to as dividend.
Capital market	A financial market in which long-term debt and equity instruments are traded is referred to as a capital market. The capital market includes the stock market and the bond market.
Fixed asset	Fixed asset, also known as property, plant, and equipment (PP&E), is a term used in accountancy for assets and property which cannot easily be converted into cash. This can be compared with current assets such as cash or bank accounts, which are described as liquid assets. In most cases, only tangible assets are referred to as fixed.
Property	Assets defined in the broadest legal sense. Property includes the unrealized receivables of a cash basis taxpayer, but not services rendered.
Accumulated depreciation	Accumulated depreciation refers to the total depreciation that has been reported as depreciation expense for the entire life of a long-term tangible asset. It is a contra-asset account.
Historical cost	In accounting terminology, historical cost describes the original cost of an asset at the time of purchase or payment as opposed to its market value
Depreciation	Depreciation is an accounting and finance term for the method of attributing the cost of an asset across the useful life of the asset. Depreciation is a reduction in the value of a currency in floating exchange rate.
Contra account	Contra account refers to an account that normally has a balance opposite to that of the other

Chapter 4. The Balance Sheet and Statement of Cash Flows

Chapter 4. The Balance Sheet and Statement of Cash Flows

	accounts in a particular category. An account whose balance is subtracted from an associated account in the financial statement.
Book value	The book value of an asset or group of assets is sometimes the price at which they were originally acquired, in many cases equal to purchase price.
Depreciation expense	Depreciation expense refers to the amount recognized as an expense in one period resulting from the periodic recognition of the used portion of the cost of a long-term tangible asset over its life.
Authority	Authority in agency law, refers to an agent's ability to affect his principal's legal relations with third parties. Also used to refer to an actor's legal power or ability to do something. In addition, sometimes used to refer to a statute, case, or other legal source that justifies a particular result.
Credit	Credit refers to a recording as positive in the balance of payments, any transaction that gives rise to a payment into the country, such as an export, the sale of an asset, or borrowing from abroad.
Vendor	A person who sells property to a vendee is a vendor. The words vendor and vendee are more commonly applied to the seller and purchaser of real estate, and the words seller and buyer are more commonly applied to the seller and purchaser of personal property.
Grant	Grant refers to an intergovernmental transfer of funds . Since the New Deal, state and local governments have become increasingly dependent upon federal grants for an almost infinite variety of programs.
Wage	The payment for the service of a unit of labor, per unit time. In trade theory, it is the only payment to labor, usually unskilled labor. In empirical work, wage data may exclude other compenzation, which must be added to get the total cost of employment.
Collateral	Property that is pledged to the lender to guarantee payment in the event that the borrower is unable to make debt payments is called collateral.
Liquidation	Liquidation refers to a process whereby the assets of a business are converted to money. The conversion may be coerced by a legal process to pay off the debt of the business, or to satisfy any other business obligation that the business has not voluntarily satisfied.
Bankruptcy	Bankruptcy is a legally declared inability or impairment of ability of an individual or organization to pay their creditors.
Principal	In agency law, one under whose direction an agent acts and for whose benefit that agent acts is a principal.
Default	In finance, default occurs when a debtor has not met its legal obligations according to the debt contract, e.g. it has not made a scheduled payment, or violated a covenant (condition) of the debt contract.
Notes payable	Notes payable refers to an obligation in the form of a written promissory note. It is a balance sheet term referring to a company's outstanding bank loans.
Trade credit	Trade credit refers to an amount that is loaned to an exporter to be repaid when the exports are paid for by the foreign importer.
Accrued expenses	Expenses that have been incurred by the end of the current accounting period but that will not be paid until a future accounting period are accrued expenses.
Accrued expense	In accrual basis accounting, accrued expense is a liability resulting from an expense for which no invoice or other official document is available yet.
Debt financing	Obtaining financing by borrowing money is debt financing.

Chapter 4. The Balance Sheet and Statement of Cash Flows

Chapter 4. The Balance Sheet and Statement of Cash Flows

Utility	Utility refers to the want-satisfying power of a good or service; the satisfaction or pleasure a consumer obtains from the consumption of a good or service.
Accrual	An accrual is an accounting event in which the transaction is recognized when the action takes place, instead of when cash is disbursed or received.
Bondholder	The individual or entity that purchases a bond, thus loaning money to the company that issued the bond is the bondholder.
Lease	A contract for the possession and use of land or other property, including goods, on one side, and a recompense of rent or other income on the other is the lease.
Net assets	Net assets refers to portion of the assets remaining after the creditors' claims have been satisfied; also called equity or residual interest.
Residual value	Residual value is one of the constituents of a leasing calculus or operation. It describes the future value of a good in terms of percentage of depreciation of its initial value.
Remainder	A remainder in property law is a future interest created in a transferee that is capable of becoming possessory upon the natural termination of a prior estate created by the same instrument.
Equity capital	Equity capital refers to money raized from within the firm or through the sale of ownership in the firm.
Contribution	In business organization law, the cash or property contributed to a business by its owners is referred to as contribution.
Charitable contributions	Charitable contributions refers to contributions that are tax deductible if made to qualified nonprofit charitable organizations. A cash basis taxpayer is entitled to a deduction solely in the year of payment.
Bottom line	The bottom line is net income on the last line of a income statement.
Profit	Profit refers to the return to the resource entrepreneurial ability; total revenue minus total cost.
Economic substance	Refers to part of a transaction that involves an activity other than the exchange of cash. Providing a service or delivering goods would be considered the economic substance of a transaction.
Contributed capital	Contributed capital is the value of funds or other consideration contributed to a company in return for an ownership interest. For instance, contributed capital increases when a person invests money in a company and received a stock certificate recognizing their right to share in the profits and losses of a company and increases or decreases in the equity value of the company.
Stockholder	A stockholder is an individual or company (including a corporation) that legally owns one or more shares of stock in a joined stock company. The shareholders are the owners of a corporation. Companies listed at the stock market strive to enhance shareholder value.
Common stock	Common stock refers to the basic, normal, voting stock issued by a corporation; called residual equity because it ranks after preferred stock for dividend and liquidation distributions.
Capital in excess of par	The amount of contributed capital less the par value of the stock is capital in excess of
Retained earnings	Cumulative earnings of a company that are not distributed to the owners and are reinvested in the business are called retained earnings.
Shares	Shares refer to an equity security, representing a shareholder's ownership of a corporation.

Go to Cram101.com for the Practice Tests for this Chapter.

Chapter 4. The Balance Sheet and Statement of Cash Flows

Chapter 4. The Balance Sheet and Statement of Cash Flows

	Shares are one of a finite number of equal portions in the capital of a company, entitling the owner to a proportion of distributed, non-reinvested profits known as dividends and to a portion of the value of the company in case of liquidation.
Bylaw	In corporation law, a document that supplements the articles of incorporation and contains less important rights, powers, and responsibilities of a corporation and its shareholders, officers, and directors is referred to as a bylaw.
Par value	The central value of a pegged exchange rate, around which the actual rate is permitted to fluctuate within set bounds is a par value.
Accumulation	The acquisition of an increasing quantity of something. The accumulation of factors, especially capital, is a primary mechanism for economic growth.
Acquisition	A company's purchase of the property and obligations of another company is an acquisition.
Fund accounting	Type of accounting used by governmental entities is referred to as fund accounting.
Deductible	The dollar sum of costs that an insured individual must pay before the insurer begins to pay is called deductible.
Fiduciary	Fiduciary refers to one who holds goods in trust for another or one who holds a position of trust and confidence.
Firm	An organization that employs resources to produce a good or service for profit and owns and operates one or more plants is referred to as a firm.
Direct method	The method of presenting the operating activities section of the statement of cash flow statement reports components of cash flows from operating activities as gross receipts and gross payments is called direct method.
Indirect method	The method of presenting the operating activities section of the statement of cash flows that adjusts net income to compute cash flows from operating activities is referred to as indirect method.
Cash flows from financing activities	Movement of funds related to the financing of the company which is reported on the cash flow statement of a company's annual report are cash flows from financing activities.
Cash flows from investing activities	Movement of funds related to the company's investments, reported on the cash flow statement of a company's annual report are cash flows from investing activities.
Cash flows from operating activities	Movement of funds related to the company's operations, reported on the cash flow statement of a company's annual report are cash flows from operating activities.
Financing activities	Cash flow activities that include obtaining cash from issuing debt and repaying the amounts borrowed and obtaining cash from stockholders and paying dividends is referred to as financing activities.
Investing activities	Investing activities refers to cash flow activities that include purchasing and disposing of investments and productive long-lived assets using cash and lending money and collecting on those loans.
Operating activities	Cash flow activities that include the cash effects of transactions that create revenues and expenses and thus enter into the determination of net income is an operating activities.
Accrual accounting	Method of accounting that records the effects of accounting events in the period in which such events occur regardless of when cash is exchanged is accrual accounting.
Financial assets	Financial assets refer to monetary claims or obligations by one party against another party.

Chapter 4. The Balance Sheet and Statement of Cash Flows

Chapter 4. The Balance Sheet and Statement of Cash Flows

	Examples are bonds, mortgages, bank loans, and equities.
Advertising	Advertising refers to paid, nonpersonal communication through various media by organizations and individuals who are in some way identified in the advertising message.
Accounts payable	A written record of all vendors to whom the business firm owes money is referred to as accounts payable.
Payables	Obligations to make future economic sacrifices, usually cash payments, are referred to as payables. Same as current liabilities.
Debt ratio	Debt ratio refers to the calculation of the total liabilities divided by the total liabilities plus capital. This results in the measurment of the debt level of the business (leverage).
Points	Loan origination fees that may be deductible as interest by a buyer of property. A seller of property who pays points reduces the selling price by the amount of the points paid for the buyer.
Financial accounting	Financial accounting is the branch of accountancy concerned with the preparation of financial statements for external decision makers, such as stockholders, suppliers, banks and government agencies. The fundamental need for financial accounting is to reduce principal-agent problem by measuring and monitoring agents' performance.
Lender	Suppliers and financial institutions that lend money to companies is referred to as a lender.
Net worth	Net worth is the total assets minus total liabilities of an individual or company
Capital structure	Capital Structure refers to the way a corporation finances itself through some combination of equity sales, equity options, bonds, and loans. Optimal capital structure refers to the particular combination that minimizes the cost of capital while maximizing the stock price.
Equity financing	Financing that consists of funds that are invested in exchange for ownership in the company is called equity financing.
Financing statement	A document, usually a multicopy form, filed in a public office serving as constructive notice to the world that a creditor claims a security interest in collateral that belongs to a certain named debtor is a financing statement.
Shareholder	A shareholder is an individual or company (including a corporation) that legally owns one or more shares of stock in a joined stock company.
Instrument	Instrument refers to an economic variable that is controlled by policy makers and can be used to influence other variables, called targets. Examples are monetary and fiscal policies used to achieve external and internal balance.
Corporation	A legal entity chartered by a state or the Federal government that is distinct and separate from the individuals who own it is a corporation. This separation gives the corporation unique powers which other legal entities lack.
Regulation	Regulation refers to restrictions state and federal laws place on business with regard to the conduct of its activities.
Subcontractor	A subcontractor is an individual or in many cases a business that signs a contract to perform part or all of the obligations of another's contract. A subcontractor is hired by a general or prime contractor to perform a specific task as part of the overall project.
Subcontract	A subcontract is a contract that assigns part of an existing contract to a different party.
Audit	An examination of the financial reports to ensure that they represent what they claim and conform with generally accepted accounting principles is referred to as audit.

Go to **Cram101.com** for the Practice Tests for this Chapter.

Chapter 4. The Balance Sheet and Statement of Cash Flows

Chapter 4. The Balance Sheet and Statement of Cash Flows

American Institute of Certified Public Accountants	With over 350,000 CPA members (in 2005), the American Institute of Certified Public Accountants is the largest CPA professional organization in the United States of America. Approximately 40% of its members are engaged in the practice of public accounting, in areas such as auditing, accounting, taxation, general business consulting, business valuation, personal financial planning and business technology.
Certified Public Accountant	Certified Public Accountant refers to an individual in the United States who have passed the Uniform Certified Public Accountant Examination and have met additional state education and experience requirements for certification as a Certified Public Accountant.
Financial management	The job of managing a firm's resources so it can meet its goals and objectives is called financial management.

Chapter 4. The Balance Sheet and Statement of Cash Flows

Chapter 5. Managerial Accounting Basics, Cost Behavior and Profit Analysis

Breakeven point	Breakeven point refers to quantity of output sold at which total revenues equal total costs, that is where the economic profit is zero.
Profit	Profit refers to the return to the resource entrepreneurial ability; total revenue minus total cost.
Points	Loan origination fees that may be deductible as interest by a buyer of property. A seller of property who pays points reduces the selling price by the amount of the points paid for the buyer.
Financial accounting	Financial accounting is the branch of accountancy concerned with the preparation of financial statements for external decision makers, such as stockholders, suppliers, banks and government agencies. The fundamental need for financial accounting is to reduce principal-agent problem by measuring and monitoring agents' performance.
Accounting	A system that collects and processes financial information about an organization and reports that information to decision makers is referred to as accounting.
Financial statement	Financial statement refers to a summary of all the transactions that have occurred over a particular period.
Managerial Accounting	Managerial accounting is the branch of accounting that uses both past and future data in providing information that management uses in conducting daily operations in planning future operations, and in developing overall business strategies.
Income statement	Income statement refers to a financial statement that presents the revenues and expenses and resulting net income or net loss of a company for a specific period of time.
Cost accounting	Cost accounting measures and reports financial and nonfinancial information relating to the cost of acquiring or consuming resources in an organization. It provides information for both management accounting and financial accounting.
Expense	In accounting, an expense represents an event in which an asset is used up or a liability is incurred. In terms of the accounting equation, expenses reduce owners' equity.
Service	Service refers to a "non tangible product" that is not embodied in a physical good and that typically effects some change in another product, person, or institution. Contrasts with good.
Variable	A variable is something measured by a number; it is used to analyze what happens to other things when the size of that number changes.
Relevant range	The range of activity within which management expects the organization to operate is called the relevant range. The range of activity over which changes in cost are of interest to management.
Fixed cost	The cost that a firm bears if it does not produce at all and that is independent of its output. The presence of a fixed cost tends to imply increasing returns to scale. Contrasts with variable cost.
Asset	An item of property, such as land, capital, money, a share in ownership, or a claim on others for future payment, such as a bond or a bank deposit is an asset.
Staffing	Staffing refers to a management function that includes hiring, motivating, and retaining the best people available to accomplish the company's objectives.
Property	Assets defined in the broadest legal sense. Property includes the unrealized receivables of a cash basis taxpayer, but not services rendered.
Variable cost	The portion of a firm or industry's cost that changes with output, in contrast to fixed cost is referred to as variable cost.

Chapter 5. Managerial Accounting Basics, Cost Behavior and Profit Analysis

Chapter 5. Managerial Accounting Basics, Cost Behavior and Profit Analysis

Cost structure	The relative proportion of an organization's fixed, variable, and mixed costs is referred to as cost structure.
Cost behavior	The relationship between cost and volume or activity is referred to as cost behavior.
Supply	Supply is the aggregate amount of any material good that can be called into being at a certain price point; it comprises one half of the equation of supply and demand. In classical economic theory, a curve representing supply is one of the factors that produce price.
Total variable Cost	The total of all costs that vary with output in the short run is called total variable cost.
Total cost	The sum of fixed cost and variable cost is referred to as total cost.
Labor	People's physical and mental talents and efforts that are used to help produce goods and services are called labor.
Average fixed Cost	Average fixed cost refers to total fixed cost divided by the number of units of output; a per-unit measure of fixed costs.
Total fixed costs	The total of all costs that do not change with output, even if output is zero is referred to as total fixed costs. Examples are rent, interest on loans, and insurance
Average cost	Average cost is equal to total cost divided by the number of goods produced (Quantity-Q). It is also equal to the sum of average variable costs (total variable costs divided by Q) plus average fixed costs (total fixed costs divided by Q).
Incentive	An incentive is any factor (financial or non-financial) that provides a motive for a particular course of action, or counts as a reason for preferring one choice to the alternatives.
Complexity	The technical sophistication of the product and hence the amount of understanding required to use it is referred to as complexity. It is the opposite of simplicity.
Slope	The slope of a line in the plane containing the x and y axes is generally represented by the letter m, and is defined as the change in the y coordinate divided by the corresponding change in the x coordinate, between two distinct points on the line.
Personnel	A collective term for all of the employees of an organization. Personnel is also commonly used to refer to the personnel management function or the organizational unit responsible for administering personnel programs.
Total revenue	Total revenue refers to the total number of dollars received by a firm from the sale of a product; equal to the total expenditures for the product produced by the firm; equal to the quantity sold multiplied by the price at which it is sold.
Revenue	Revenue is a U.S. business term for the amount of money that a company receives from its activities, mostly from sales of products and/or services to customers.
Net income	Net income is equal to the income that a firm has after subtracting costs and expenses from the total revenue. Expenses will typically include tax expense.
Profit and loss statement	Profit and loss statement refers to another term for the income statement.
Contribution margin	A company's contribution margin can be expressed as the percentage of each sale that remains after the variable costs are subtracted. In simplest terms, the contribution margin is total revenue minus total variable cost.
Contribution	In business organization law, the cash or property contributed to a business by its owners is referred to as contribution.

Chapter 5. Managerial Accounting Basics, Cost Behavior and Profit Analysis

Chapter 5. Managerial Accounting Basics, Cost Behavior and Profit Analysis

Margin	A deposit by a buyer in stocks with a seller or a stockbroker, as security to cover fluctuations in the market in reference to stocks that the buyer has purchased but for which he has not paid is a margin. Commodities are also traded on margin.
Context	The effect of the background under which a message often takes on more and richer meaning is a context. Context is especially important in cross-cultural interactions because some cultures are said to be high context or low context.
Operating leverage	Effects that fixed costs have on changes in operating income as changes occur in units sold and hence in contribution margin are called operating leverage.
Leverage	Leverage is using given resources in such a way that the potential positive or negative outcome is magnified. In finance, this generally refers to borrowing.
Market	A market is, as defined in economics, a social arrangement that allows buyers and sellers to discover information and carry out a voluntary exchange of goods or services.
Bottom line	The bottom line is net income on the last line of a income statement.
Top line	Top line refers to the total revenues or sales mentioned in the income statement. This refers to the fact that the total revenues collected by a company appears at the top of the income statement. This is in contrast to the net profit that is calculated after subtracting the net expenses. Since this forms the last line of the income statement, it is generally referred to the bottom line.
Earnings before interest and taxes	Income from operations before subtracting interest expense and income taxes is an earnings before interest and taxes.
Degree of operating leverage	Contribution margin divided by operating income at any given level of sales is a degree of operating leverage.
Interest expense	The cost a business incurs to borrow money. With respect to bonds payable, the interest expense is calculated by multiplying the market rate of interest by the carrying value of the bonds on the date of the payment.
Interest	In finance and economics, interest is the price paid by a borrower for the use of a lender's money. In other words, interest is the amount of paid to "rent" money for a period of time.
Industry	A group of firms that produce identical or similar products is an industry. It is also used specifically to refer to an area of economic production focused on manufacturing which involves large amounts of capital investment before any profit can be realized, also called "heavy industry".
Economies of scale	In economics, returns to scale and economies of scale are related terms that describe what happens as the scale of production increases. They are different terms and not to be used interchangeably.
Economics	The social science dealing with the use of scarce resources to obtain the maximum satisfaction of society's virtually unlimited economic wants is an economics.
Economy	The income, expenditures, and resources that affect the cost of running a business and household are called an economy.
Fixed asset	Fixed asset, also known as property, plant, and equipment (PP&E), is a term used in accountancy for assets and property which cannot easily be converted into cash. This can be compared with current assets such as cash or bank accounts, which are described as liquid assets. In most cases, only tangible assets are referred to as fixed.
Investment	Investment refers to spending for the production and accumulation of capital and additions to

Chapter 5. Managerial Accounting Basics, Cost Behavior and Profit Analysis

Chapter 5. Managerial Accounting Basics, Cost Behavior and Profit Analysis

	inventories. In a financial sense, buying an asset with the expectation of making a return.
Market share	That fraction of an industry's output accounted for by an individual firm or group of firms is called market share.
Core	A core is the set of feasible allocations in an economy that cannot be improved upon by subset of the set of the economy's consumers (a coalition). In construction, when the force in an element is within a certain center section, the core, the element will only be under compression.
Discount	The difference between the face value of a bond and its selling price, when a bond is sold for less than its face value it's referred to as a discount.
Marginal cost	Marginal cost refers to the increase in cost that accompanies a unit increase in output; the partial derivative of the cost function with respect to output.
Contract	A contract is a "promise" or an "agreement" that is enforced or recognized by the law. In the civil law, a contract is considered to be part of the general law of obligations.
Recovery	Characterized by rizing output, falling unemployment, rizing profits, and increasing economic activity following a decline is a recovery.
Coalition	An informal alliance among managers who support a specific goal is called coalition.
Insurance	Insurance refers to a system by which individuals can reduce their exposure to risk of large losses by spreading the risks among a large number of persons.
Premium	Premium refers to the fee charged by an insurance company for an insurance policy. The rate of losses must be relatively predictable: In order to set the premium (prices) insurers must be able to estimate them accurately.
Management	Management characterizes the process of leading and directing all or part of an organization, often a business, through the deployment and manipulation of resources. Early twentieth-century management writer Mary Parker Follett defined management as "the art of getting things done through people."
Financial perspective	Financial perspective is one of the four standard perspectives used with the Balanced Scorecard. Financial perspective measures inform an organization whether strategy execution, which is detailed through measures in the other three perspectives, is leading to improved bottom line results.
Financial risk	The risk related to the inability of the firm to meet its debt obligations as they come due is called financial risk.
Lease	A contract for the possession and use of land or other property, including goods, on one side, and a recompense of rent or other income on the other is the lease.
Operation	A standardized method or technique that is performed repetitively, often on different materials resulting in different finished goods is called an operation.
Marginal analysis	The comparison of marginal benefits and marginal costs, usually for decision making is a marginal analysis.
Average variable cost	A firm's total variable cost divided by output is called average variable cost.
Management accounting	Management accounting measures and reports financial and nonfinancial information that helps managers make decisions to fulfill the goals of an organization. It focuses on internal reporting.
Quality improvement	Quality is inversely proportional to variability thus quality Improvement is the reduction of variability in products and processes.

Go to **Cram101.com** for the Practice Tests for this Chapter.

Chapter 5. Managerial Accounting Basics, Cost Behavior and Profit Analysis

Chapter 5. Managerial Accounting Basics, Cost Behavior and Profit Analysis

Financial management	The job of managing a firm's resources so it can meet its goals and objectives is called financial management.
Productivity	Productivity refers to the total output of goods and services in a given period of time divided by work hours.
Journal	Book of original entry, in which transactions are recorded in a general ledger system, is referred to as a journal.

Chapter 6. Cost Allocation

Cost driver	Cost driver refers to a factor related to an activity that changes the volume or characteristics of that activity, and in doing so changes its costs. An activity can have more than one cost driver.
Overhead cost	An expenses of operating a business over and above the direct costs of producing a product is an overhead cost. They can include utilities (eg, electricity, telephone), advertizing and marketing, and any other costs not billed directly to the client or included in the price of the product.
Allocate	Allocate refers to the assignment of income for various tax purposes. A multistate corporation's nonbusiness income usually is distributed to the state where the nonbusiness assets are located; it is not apportioned with the rest of the entity's income.
Revenue	Revenue is a U.S. business term for the amount of money that a company receives from its activities, mostly from sales of products and/or services to customers.
Service	Service refers to a "non tangible product" that is not embodied in a physical good and that typically effects some change in another product, person, or institution. Contrasts with good.
Cost structure	The relative proportion of an organization's fixed, variable, and mixed costs is referred to as cost structure.
Supply	Supply is the aggregate amount of any material good that can be called into being at a certain price point; it comprises one half of the equation of supply and demand. In classical economic theory, a curve representing supply is one of the factors that produce price.
Direct cost	A direct cost is a cost that can be identified specifically with a particular sponsored project, an instructional activity, or any other institutional activity, or that can be directly assigned to such activities relatively easily with a high degree of accuracy.
Indirect cost	Indirect cost refers to a cost that cannot be traced to a particular department.
Cost allocation	Cost allocation refers to the process of assigning costs in a cost pool to the appropriate cost objects.
Assignment	A transfer of property or some right or interest is referred to as assignment.
Market	A market is, as defined in economics, a social arrangement that allows buyers and sellers to discover information and carry out a voluntary exchange of goods or services.
Administrator	Administrator refers to the personal representative appointed by a probate court to settle the estate of a deceased person who died.
Management	Management characterizes the process of leading and directing all or part of an organization, often a business, through the deployment and manipulation of resources. Early twentieth-century management writer Mary Parker Follett defined management as "the art of getting things done through people."
Personnel	A collective term for all of the employees of an organization. Personnel is also commonly used to refer to the personnel management function or the organizational unit responsible for administering personnel programs.
Contract	A contract is a "promise" or an "agreement" that is enforced or recognized by the law. In the civil law, a contract is considered to be part of the general law of obligations.
Accounting	A system that collects and processes financial information about an organization and reports that information to decision makers is referred to as accounting.
Managerial Accounting	Managerial accounting is the branch of accounting that uses both past and future data in providing information that management uses in conducting daily operations in planning future

Chapter 6. Cost Allocation

Chapter 6. Cost Allocation

	operations, and in developing overall business strategies.
Cost pool	Cost pool refers to a group of specific indirect costs created by the same cost drivers; the total cost pool amount is usually allocated to specific products or cost centers on the basis of estimated production over a period of time.
Total cost	The sum of fixed cost and variable cost is referred to as total cost.
Negotiation	Negotiation is the process whereby interested parties resolve disputes, agree upon courses of action, bargain for individual or collective advantage, and/or attempt to craft outcomes which serve their mutual interests.
Management system	A management system is the framework of processes and procedures used to ensure that an organization can fulfill all tasks required to achieve its objectives.
Cost management	The approaches and activities of managers in short-run and long-run planning and control decisions that increase value for customers and lower costs of products and services are called cost management.
Correlation	A correlation is the measure of the extent to which two economic or statistical variables move together, normalized so that its values range from -1 to +1. It is defined as the covariance of the two variables divided by the square root of the product of their variances.
Variable	A variable is something measured by a number; it is used to analyze what happens to other things when the size of that number changes.
Labor	People's physical and mental talents and efforts that are used to help produce goods and services are called labor.
Direct method	The method of presenting the operating activities section of the statement of cash flow statement reports components of cash flows from operating activities as gross receipts and gross payments is called direct method.
Compromise	Compromise occurs when the interaction is moderately important to meeting goals and the goals are neither completely compatible nor completely incompatible.
Complexity	The technical sophistication of the product and hence the amount of understanding required to use it is referred to as complexity. It is the opposite of simplicity.
Human resources	Human resources refers to the individuals within the firm, and to the portion of the firm's organization that deals with hiring, firing, training, and other personnel issues.
Administration	Administration refers to the management and direction of the affairs of governments and institutions; a collective term for all policymaking officials of a government; the execution and implementation of public policy.
Rational pricing	Rational pricing is the assumption in financial economics that asset prices (and hence asset pricing models) will reflect the arbitrage-free price of the asset as any deviation from this price will be "arbitraged away".
Preparation	Preparation refers to usually the first stage in the creative process. It includes education and formal training.
Tying	Tying is the practice of making the sale of one good (the tying good) to the de facto or de jure customer conditional on the purchase of a second distinctive good.
Incentive system	An incentive system refers to plans in which employees can earn additional compenzation in return for certain types of performance.
Incentive	An incentive is any factor (financial or non-financial) that provides a motive for a particular course of action, or counts as a reason for preferring one choice to the alternatives.

Go to Cram101.com for the Practice Tests for this Chapter.

Chapter 6. Cost Allocation

Chapter 6. Cost Allocation

Long run	In economic models, the long run time frame assumes no fixed factors of production. Firms can enter or leave the marketplace, and the cost (and availability) of land, labor, raw materials, and capital goods can be assumed to vary.
Direct labor	The earnings of employees who work directly on the products being manufactured are direct labor.
Cost accounting	Cost accounting measures and reports financial and nonfinancial information relating to the cost of acquiring or consuming resources in an organization. It provides information for both management accounting and financial accounting.
Gain	In finance, gain is a profit or an increase in value of an investment such as a stock or bond. Gain is calculated by fair market value or the proceeds from the sale of the investment minus the sum of the purchase price and all costs associated with it.
Medicare	Medicare refers to federal program that is financed by payroll taxes and provides for compulsory hospital insurance for senior citizens and low-cost voluntary insurance to help older Americans pay physicians' fees.
Activity based costing	A control system that identifies the various activities needed to provide a product and allocates costs accordingly is an activity based costing.
Industry	A group of firms that produce identical or similar products is an industry. It is also used specifically to refer to an area of economic production focused on manufacturing which involves large amounts of capital investment before any profit can be realized, also called "heavy industry".
Foundation	A Foundation is a type of philanthropic organization set up by either individuals or institutions as a legal entity (either as a corporation or trust) with the purpose of distributing grants to support causes in line with the goals of the foundation.
Administrative cost	An administrative cost is all executive, organizational, and clerical costs associated with the general management of an organization rather than with manufacturing, marketing, or selling
Accounting information system	The system of collecting and processing transaction data and communicating financial information to interested parties is called the accounting information system.
Information system	An information system is a system whether automated or manual, that comprises people, machines, and/or methods organized to collect, process, transmit, and disseminate data that represent user information.
Consideration	Consideration in contract law, a basic requirement for an enforceable agreement under traditional contract principles, defined in this text as legal value, bargained for and given in exchange for an act or promise. In corporation law, cash or property contributed to a corporation in exchange for shares, or a promise to contribute such cash or property.
Total revenue	Total revenue refers to the total number of dollars received by a firm from the sale of a product; equal to the total expenditures for the product produced by the firm; equal to the quantity sold multiplied by the price at which it is sold.
Allocation scheme	An allocation scheme is an agreement in which competitors divide markets among themselves.
Devise	In a will, a gift of real property is called a devise.
Journal	Book of original entry, in which transactions are recorded in a general ledger system, is referred to as a journal.
Investment	Investment refers to spending for the production and accumulation of capital and additions to

Chapter 6. Cost Allocation

Chapter 6. Cost Allocation

	inventories. In a financial sense, buying an asset with the expectation of making a return.
Capital	Capital generally refers to financial wealth, especially that used to start or maintain a business. In classical economics, capital is one of four factors of production, the others being land and labor and entrepreneurship.
Adoption	In corporation law, a corporation's acceptance of a pre-incorporation contract by action of its board of directors, by which the corporation becomes liable on the contract, is referred to as adoption.
Financial management	The job of managing a firm's resources so it can meet its goals and objectives is called financial management.
Controlling	A management function that involves determining whether or not an organization is progressing toward its goals and objectives, and taking corrective action if it is not is called controlling.

Chapter 6. Cost Allocation

Chapter 7. Pricing and Service Decisions

Service	Service refers to a "non tangible product" that is not embodied in a physical good and that typically effects some change in another product, person, or institution. Contrasts with good.
Accounting	A system that collects and processes financial information about an organization and reports that information to decision makers is referred to as accounting.
Managerial Accounting	Managerial accounting is the branch of accounting that uses both past and future data in providing information that management uses in conducting daily operations in planning future operations, and in developing overall business strategies.
Coalition	An informal alliance among managers who support a specific goal is called coalition.
Discount	The difference between the face value of a bond and its selling price, when a bond is sold for less than its face value it's referred to as a discount.
Revenue	Revenue is a U.S. business term for the amount of money that a company receives from its activities, mostly from sales of products and/or services to customers.
Market	A market is, as defined in economics, a social arrangement that allows buyers and sellers to discover information and carry out a voluntary exchange of goods or services.
Economic theory	Economic theory refers to a statement of a cause-effect relationship; when accepted by all economists, an economic principle.
Perfectly competitive market	Exists when there is a homogeneous product and where no individual buyers or sellers can affect those prices by their own actions are referred to as perfectly competitive market.
Competitive market	A market in which no buyer or seller has market power is called a competitive market.
Price taker	Price taker refers to an economic entity that is too small relative to a market to affect its price, and that therefore must take that price as given in making its own decisions. Applies to all buyers in sellers in markets that are perfectly competitive.
Perfectly competitive	Perfectly competitive is an economic agent, group of agents, model or analysis that is characterized by perfect competition. Contrasts with imperfectly competitive.
Market power	The ability of a single economic actor to have a substantial influence on market prices is market power.
Cost structure	The relative proportion of an organization's fixed, variable, and mixed costs is referred to as cost structure.
Financial perspective	Financial perspective is one of the four standard perspectives used with the Balanced Scorecard. Financial perspective measures inform an organization whether strategy execution, which is detailed through measures in the other three perspectives, is leading to improved bottom line results.
Market dominance	Market dominance is a measure of the strength of a brand, product, service, or firm, relative to competitive offerings. There is often a geographic element to the competitive landscape. In defining market dominance, you must see to what extent a product, brand, or firm controls a product category in a given geographic area.
Market share	That fraction of an industry's output accounted for by an individual firm or group of firms is called market share.
Shares	Shares refer to an equity security, representing a shareholder's ownership of a corporation. Shares are one of a finite number of equal portions in the capital of a company, entitling the owner to a proportion of distributed, non-reinvested profits known as dividends and to a

Chapter 7. Pricing and Service Decisions

Chapter 7. Pricing and Service Decisions

	portion of the value of the company in case of liquidation.
Long run	In economic models, the long run time frame assumes no fixed factors of production. Firms can enter or leave the marketplace, and the cost (and availability) of land, labor, raw materials, and capital goods can be assumed to vary.
Profit	Profit refers to the return to the resource entrepreneurial ability; total revenue minus total cost.
Asset	An item of property, such as land, capital, money, a share in ownership, or a claim on others for future payment, such as a bond or a bank deposit is an asset.
Investment	Investment refers to spending for the production and accumulation of capital and additions to inventories. In a financial sense, buying an asset with the expectation of making a return.
Equity	Equity is the name given to the set of legal principles, in countries following the English common law tradition, which supplement strict rules of law where their application would operate harshly, so as to achieve what is sometimes referred to as "natural justice."
Marginal cost	Marginal cost refers to the increase in cost that accompanies a unit increase in output; the partial derivative of the cost function with respect to output.
Economics	The social science dealing with the use of scarce resources to obtain the maximum satisfaction of society's virtually unlimited economic wants is an economics.
Personnel	A collective term for all of the employees of an organization. Personnel is also commonly used to refer to the personnel management function or the organizational unit responsible for administering personnel programs.
Overtime	Overtime is the amount of time someone works beyond normal working hours.
Labor	People's physical and mental talents and efforts that are used to help produce goods and services are called labor.
Utility	Utility refers to the want-satisfying power of a good or service; the satisfaction or pleasure a consumer obtains from the consumption of a good or service.
Expense	In accounting, an expense represents an event in which an asset is used up or a liability is incurred. In terms of the accounting equation, expenses reduce owners' equity.
Supply	Supply is the aggregate amount of any material good that can be called into being at a certain price point; it comprises one half of the equation of supply and demand. In classical economic theory, a curve representing supply is one of the factors that produce price.
Overhead cost	An expenses of operating a business over and above the direct costs of producing a product is an overhead cost. They can include utilities (eg, electricity, telephone), advertizing and marketing, and any other costs not billed directly to the client or included in the price of the product.
Medicare	Medicare refers to federal program that is financed by payroll taxes and provides for compulsory hospital insurance for senior citizens and low-cost voluntary insurance to help older Americans pay physicians' fees.
Fixed cost	The cost that a firm bears if it does not produce at all and that is independent of its output. The presence of a fixed cost tends to imply increasing returns to scale. Contrasts with variable cost.
Fund	Independent accounting entity with a self-balancing set of accounts segregated for the purposes of carrying on specific activities is referred to as a fund.
Pricing strategy	The process in which the price of a product can be determined and is decided upon is a pricing strategy.

Chapter 7. Pricing and Service Decisions

Chapter 7. Pricing and Service Decisions

Target costing	Target costing refers to designing a product so that it satisfies customers and meets the profit margins desired by the firm.
Management	Management characterizes the process of leading and directing all or part of an organization, often a business, through the deployment and manipulation of resources. Early twentieth-century management writer Mary Parker Follett defined management as "the art of getting things done through people."
Target cost	The projected long-run product cost that will enable a firm to enter and remain in the market for the product and compete successfully with the firm's competitors is referred to as target cost.
Total variable Cost	The total of all costs that vary with output in the short run is called total variable cost.
Variable cost	The portion of a firm or industry's cost that changes with output, in contrast to fixed cost is referred to as variable cost.
Total revenue	Total revenue refers to the total number of dollars received by a firm from the sale of a product; equal to the total expenditures for the product produced by the firm; equal to the quantity sold multiplied by the price at which it is sold.
Total cost	The sum of fixed cost and variable cost is referred to as total cost.
Variable	A variable is something measured by a number; it is used to analyze what happens to other things when the size of that number changes.
Consideration	Consideration in contract law, a basic requirement for an enforceable agreement under traditional contract principles, defined in this text as legal value, bargained for and given in exchange for an act or promise. In corporation law, cash or property contributed to a corporation in exchange for shares, or a promise to contribute such cash or property.
Gain	In finance, gain is a profit or an increase in value of an investment such as a stock or bond. Gain is calculated by fair market value or the proceeds from the sale of the investment minus the sum of the purchase price and all costs associated with it.
Net income	Net income is equal to the income that a firm has after subtracting costs and expenses from the total revenue. Expenses will typically include tax expense.
Marketing	Promoting and selling products or services to customers, or prospective customers, is referred to as marketing.
Conversion	Conversion refers to any distinct act of dominion wrongfully exerted over another's personal property in denial of or inconsistent with his rights therein. That tort committed by a person who deals with chattels not belonging to him in a manner that is inconsistent with the ownership of the lawful owner.
Bottom line	The bottom line is net income on the last line of a income statement.
Contribution margin	A company's contribution margin can be expressed as the percentage of each sale that remains after the variable costs are subtracted. In simplest terms, the contribution margin is total revenue minus total variable cost.
Contribution	In business organization law, the cash or property contributed to a business by its owners is referred to as contribution.
Margin	A deposit by a buyer in stocks with a seller or a stockbroker, as security to cover fluctuations in the market in reference to stocks that the buyer has purchased but for which he has not paid is a margin. Commodities are also traded on margin.
Premium	Premium refers to the fee charged by an insurance company for an insurance policy. The rate

Chapter 7. Pricing and Service Decisions

Chapter 7. Pricing and Service Decisions

	of losses must be relatively predictable: In order to set the premium (prices) insurers must be able to estimate them accurately.
Big Business	Big business is usually used as a pejorative reference to the significant economic and political power which large and powerful corporations (especially multinational corporations), are capable of wielding.
Bid	A bid price is a price offered by a buyer when he/she buys a good. In the context of stock trading on a stock exchange, the bid price is the highest price a buyer of a stock is willing to pay for a share of that given stock.
Specialist	A specialist is a trader who makes a market in one or several stocks and holds the limit order book for those stocks.
Administration	Administration refers to the management and direction of the affairs of governments and institutions; a collective term for all policymaking officials of a government; the execution and implementation of public policy.
Contract	A contract is a "promise" or an "agreement" that is enforced or recognized by the law. In the civil law, a contract is considered to be part of the general law of obligations.
Copayment	The percentage of costs that an insured individual pays while the insurer pays the remainder is called a copayment.
Value system	A value system refers to how an individual or a group of individuals organize their ethical or ideological values. A well-defined value system is a moral code.
Profit margin	Profit margin is a measure of profitability. It is calculated using a formula and written as a percentage or a number. Profit margin = Net income before tax and interest / Revenue.
Case analysis	Case analysis is one of the most general and applicable methods of analytical thinking, depending only on the division of a problem, decision or situation into a sufficient number of separate cases.
Management system	A management system is the framework of processes and procedures used to ensure that an organization can fulfill all tasks required to achieve its objectives.
Administrative cost	An administrative cost is all executive, organizational, and clerical costs associated with the general management of an organization rather than with manufacturing, marketing, or selling
Quality assurance	Those activities associated with assuring the quality of a product or service is called quality assurance.
Verification	Verification refers to the final stage of the creative process where the validity or truthfulness of the insight is determined. The feedback portion of communication in which the receiver sends a message to the source indicating receipt of the message and the degree to which he or she understood the message.
Net loss	Net loss refers to the amount by which expenses exceed revenues. The difference between income received and expenses, when expenses are greater.
Short run	Short run refers to a period of time that permits an increase or decrease in current production volume with existing capacity, but one that is too short to permit enlargement of that capacity itself (eg, the building of new plants, training of additional workers, etc.).
Demographic	A demographic is a term used in marketing and broadcasting, to describe a demographic grouping or a market segment.
Scenario analysis	Scenario analysis is a process of analyzing possible future events by considering alternative possible outcomes. The analysis is designed to allow improved decision-making by allowing

Chapter 7. Pricing and Service Decisions

Chapter 7. Pricing and Service Decisions

	more complete consideration of outcomes and their implications.
Sensitivity analysis	A what-if technique that managers use to examine how a result will change if the original predicted data are not achieved or if an underlying assumption changes is sensitivity analysis.
Journal	Book of original entry, in which transactions are recorded in a general ledger system, is referred to as a journal.
Financial management	The job of managing a firm's resources so it can meet its goals and objectives is called financial management.
Relevant cost	A relevant cost refers to expected future costs that differ among alternative courses of action being considered. A cost that will be affected by taking a particular decision.
Policy	Similar to a script in that a policy can be a less than completely rational decision-making method. Involves the use of a pre-existing set of decision steps for any problem that presents itself.
Yield	The interest rate that equates a future value or an annuity to a given present value is a yield.
Markup	Markup is a term used in marketing to indicate how much the price of a product is above the cost of producing and distributing the product.

Chapter 7. Pricing and Service Decisions

Chapter 8. Planning and Budgeting

Budget	Budget refers to an account, usually for a year, of the planned expenditures and the expected receipts of an entity. For a government, the receipts are tax revenues.
Flexible budget	A budget developed using budgeted revenues and budgeted costs based on the actual output level in the budget period is referred to as flexible budget.
Static budget	Budget based on a single level of output is a static budget.
Variance analysis	In budgeting or (management accounting in general) variance analysis is a tool of budgetary control by evaluation of performance by means of variances between budgeted, planned or standard amount and the actual amount incurred/sold. Variance analysis can be carried for both costs and revenues.
Variance	Variance refers to a measure of how much an economic or statistical variable varies across values or observations. Its calculation is the same as that of the covariance, being the covariance of the variable with itself.
Cash budget	A projection of anticipated cash flows, usually over a one to two year period is called a cash budget.
Service	Service refers to a "non tangible product" that is not embodied in a physical good and that typically effects some change in another product, person, or institution. Contrasts with good.
Accounting	A system that collects and processes financial information about an organization and reports that information to decision makers is referred to as accounting.
Managerial Accounting	Managerial accounting is the branch of accounting that uses both past and future data in providing information that management uses in conducting daily operations in planning future operations, and in developing overall business strategies.
Mission statement	Mission statement refers to an outline of the fundamental purposes of an organization.
Scope	Scope of a project is the sum total of all projects products and their requirements or features.
Strategic plan	The formal document that presents the ways and means by which a strategic goal will be achieved is a strategic plan. A long-term flexible plan that does not regulate activities but rather outlines the means to achieve certain results, and provides the means to alter the course of action should the desired ends change.
Time horizon	A time horizon is a fixed point of time in the future at which point certain processes will be evaluated or assumed to end. It is necessary in an accounting, finance or risk management regime to assign such a fixed horizon time so that alternatives can be evaluated for performance over the same period of time.
Financial plan	The financial plan section of a business plan consists of three financial statements (the income statement, the cash flow projection, and the balance sheet) and a brief analysis of these three statements.
Remainder	A remainder in property law is a future interest created in a transferee that is capable of becoming possessory upon the natural termination of a prior estate created by the same instrument.
Capital budget	A long-term budget that shows planned acquisition and disposal of capital assets, such as land, building, and equipment is a capital budget. Also a separate budget used by state governments for items such as new construction, major renovations, and acquisition of physical property.
Investment	Investment refers to spending for the production and accumulation of capital and additions to

Chapter 8. Planning and Budgeting

Chapter 8. Planning and Budgeting

	inventories. In a financial sense, buying an asset with the expectation of making a return.
Capital	Capital generally refers to financial wealth, especially that used to start or maintain a business. In classical economics, capital is one of four factors of production, the others being land and labor and entrepreneurship.
Asset	An item of property, such as land, capital, money, a share in ownership, or a claim on others for future payment, such as a bond or a bank deposit is an asset.
Working capital management	Working capital management refers to the financing and management of the current assets of the firm. The financial manager determines the mix between temporary and permanent 'current assets' and the nature of the financing arrangement.
Working capital	The dollar difference between total current assets and total current liabilities is called working capital.
Management	Management characterizes the process of leading and directing all or part of an organization, often a business, through the deployment and manipulation of resources. Early twentieth-century management writer Mary Parker Follett defined management as "the art of getting things done through people."
Current liability	Current liability refers to a debt that can reasonably be expected to be paid from existing current assets or through the creation of other current liabilities, within one year or the operating cycle, whichever is longer.
Human resources	Human resources refers to the individuals within the firm, and to the portion of the firm's organization that deals with hiring, firing, training, and other personnel issues.
Current asset	A current asset is an asset on the balance sheet which is expected to be sold or otherwise used up in the near future, usually within one year.
Liability	A liability is a present obligation of the enterprise arizing from past events, the settlement of which is expected to result in an outflow from the enterprise of resources embodying economic benefits.
Operation	A standardized method or technique that is performed repetitively, often on different materials resulting in different finished goods is called an operation.
Contract	A contract is a "promise" or an "agreement" that is enforced or recognized by the law. In the civil law, a contract is considered to be part of the general law of obligations.
Capital expenditures	Major investments in long-term assets such as land, buildings, equipment, or research and development are referred to as capital expenditures.
Capital expenditure	A substantial expenditure that is used by a company to acquire or upgrade physical assets such as equipment, property, industrial buildings, including those which improve the quality and life of an asset is referred to as a capital expenditure.
Analyst	Analyst refers to a person or tool with a primary function of information analysis, generally with a more limited, practical and short term set of goals than a researcher.
Financial statement	Financial statement refers to a summary of all the transactions that have occurred over a particular period.
Fund	Independent accounting entity with a self-balancing set of accounts segregated for the purposes of carrying on specific activities is referred to as a fund.
Board of directors	The group of individuals elected by the stockholders of a corporation to oversee its operations is a board of directors.
Committee	A long-lasting, sometimes permanent team in the organization structure created to deal with tasks that recur regularly is the committee.

Go to Cram101.com for the Practice Tests for this Chapter.

Chapter 8. Planning and Budgeting

Chapter 8. Planning and Budgeting

Allocate	Allocate refers to the assignment of income for various tax purposes. A multistate corporation's nonbusiness income usually is distributed to the state where the nonbusiness assets are located; it is not apportioned with the rest of the entity's income.
Control process	A process involving gathering processed data, analyzing processed data, and using this information to make adjustments to the process is a control process.
Master budget	Master budget refers to expression of management's operating and financial plans for a specified period and comprises a set of budgeted financial statements. Also called pro forma statements.
Preference	The act of a debtor in paying or securing one or more of his creditors in a manner more favorable to them than to other creditors or to the exclusion of such other creditors is a preference. In the absence of statute, a preference is perfectly good, but to be legal it must be bona fide, and not a mere subterfuge of the debtor to secure a future benefit to himself or to prevent the application of his property to his debts.
Operating budget	An operating budget is the annual budget of an activity stated in terms of Budget Classification Code, functional/subfunctional categories and cost accounts. It contains estimates of the total value of resources required for the performance of the operation including reimbursable work or services for others.
Expense budget	A budget that outlines the anticipated and actual expenses for each responsibility center is referred to as expense budget.
Revenue	Revenue is a U.S. business term for the amount of money that a company receives from its activities, mostly from sales of products and/or services to customers.
Expense	In accounting, an expense represents an event in which an asset is used up or a liability is incurred. In terms of the accounting equation, expenses reduce owners' equity.
Ancillary	An ancillary receiver is a receiver who has been appointed in aid of, and in subordination to, the primary receiver.
Consideration	Consideration in contract law, a basic requirement for an enforceable agreement under traditional contract principles, defined in this text as legal value, bargained for and given in exchange for an act or promise. In corporation law, cash or property contributed to a corporation in exchange for shares, or a promise to contribute such cash or property.
Competitor	Other organizations in the same industry or type of business that provide a good or service to the same set of customers is referred to as a competitor.
Marketing	Promoting and selling products or services to customers, or prospective customers, is referred to as marketing.
Market share	That fraction of an industry's output accounted for by an individual firm or group of firms is called market share.
Market	A market is, as defined in economics, a social arrangement that allows buyers and sellers to discover information and carry out a voluntary exchange of goods or services.
Interest income	Interest income refers to payments of income to those who supply the economy with capital.
Interest	In finance and economics, interest is the price paid by a borrower for the use of a lender's money. In other words, interest is the amount of paid to "rent" money for a period of time.
Lease	A contract for the possession and use of land or other property, including goods, on one side, and a recompense of rent or other income on the other is the lease.
Revenue budget	A budget that identifies the forecasted and actual revenues of the organization is a revenue budget.

Chapter 8. Planning and Budgeting

Chapter 8. Planning and Budgeting

Fringe benefits	The rewards other than wages that employees receive from their employers and that include pensions, medical and dental insurance, paid vacations, and sick leaves are referred to as fringe benefits.
Fringe benefit	Benefits such as sick-leave pay, vacation pay, pension plans, and health plans that represent additional compenzation to employees beyond base wages is a fringe benefit.
Labor	People's physical and mental talents and efforts that are used to help produce goods and services are called labor.
Wage	The payment for the service of a unit of labor, per unit time. In trade theory, it is the only payment to labor, usually unskilled labor. In empirical work, wage data may exclude other compenzation, which must be added to get the total cost of employment.
Depreciation	Depreciation is an accounting and finance term for the method of attributing the cost of an asset across the useful life of the asset. Depreciation is a reduction in the value of a currency in floating exchange rate.
Utility	Utility refers to the want-satisfying power of a good or service; the satisfaction or pleasure a consumer obtains from the consumption of a good or service.
Supply	Supply is the aggregate amount of any material good that can be called into being at a certain price point; it comprises one half of the equation of supply and demand. In classical economic theory, a curve representing supply is one of the factors that produce price.
Variable	A variable is something measured by a number; it is used to analyze what happens to other things when the size of that number changes.
Accrual accounting	Method of accounting that records the effects of accounting events in the period in which such events occur regardless of when cash is exchanged is accrual accounting.
Accounting method	Accounting method refers to the method under which income and expenses are determined for tax purposes. Important accounting methods include the cash basis and the accrual basis.
Income statement	Income statement refers to a financial statement that presents the revenues and expenses and resulting net income or net loss of a company for a specific period of time.
Accrual	An accrual is an accounting event in which the transaction is recognized when the action takes place, instead of when cash is disbursed or received.
Cash flow	In finance, cash flow refers to the amounts of cash being received and spent by a business during a defined period of time, sometimes tied to a specific project. Most of the time they are being used to determine gaps in the liquid position of a company.
Statement of cash flow	Reports inflows and outflows of cash during the accounting period in the categories of operating, investing, and financing is a statement of cash flow.
Budget process	Budget process refers to the total system a jurisdiction uses to make decisions on government spending needs and how to pay for them. The main difference between federal and state and local budges processes is that the state and local jurisdictions must have balanced budgets each year.
Contribution	In business organization law, the cash or property contributed to a business by its owners is referred to as contribution.
Senior management	Senior management is generally a team of individuals at the highest level of organizational management who have the day-to-day responsibilities of managing a corporation.
Compromise	Compromise occurs when the interaction is moderately important to meeting goals and the goals are neither completely compatible nor completely incompatible.
Aggregation	Aggregation refers to the combining of two or more things into a single category. Data on

Chapter 8. Planning and Budgeting

Chapter 8. Planning and Budgeting

	international trade necessarily aggregate goods and services into manageable groups.
Negotiation	Negotiation is the process whereby interested parties resolve disputes, agree upon courses of action, bargain for individual or collective advantage, and/or attempt to craft outcomes which serve their mutual interests.
Variable cost	The portion of a firm or industry's cost that changes with output, in contrast to fixed cost is referred to as variable cost.
Total revenue	Total revenue refers to the total number of dollars received by a firm from the sale of a product; equal to the total expenditures for the product produced by the firm; equal to the quantity sold multiplied by the price at which it is sold.
Average cost	Average cost is equal to total cost divided by the number of goods produced (Quantity-Q). It is also equal to the sum of average variable costs (total variable costs divided by Q) plus average fixed costs (total fixed costs divided by Q).
Productivity	Productivity refers to the total output of goods and services in a given period of time divided by work hours.
Total variable Cost	The total of all costs that vary with output in the short run is called total variable cost.
Fixed cost	The cost that a firm bears if it does not produce at all and that is independent of its output. The presence of a fixed cost tends to imply increasing returns to scale. Contrasts with variable cost.
Profit	Profit refers to the return to the resource entrepreneurial ability; total revenue minus total cost.
Controlling	A management function that involves determining whether or not an organization is progressing toward its goals and objectives, and taking corrective action if it is not is called controlling.
Controllable cost	Any cost that is primarily subject to the influence of a given responsibility center manager for a given period is a controllable cost.
Cost variance	The difference between the actual and budgeted cost of work performed is called cost variance.
Gain	In finance, gain is a profit or an increase in value of an investment such as a stock or bond. Gain is calculated by fair market value or the proceeds from the sale of the investment minus the sum of the purchase price and all costs associated with it.
Profit and loss statement	Profit and loss statement refers to another term for the income statement.
Contribution margin	A company's contribution margin can be expressed as the percentage of each sale that remains after the variable costs are subtracted. In simplest terms, the contribution margin is total revenue minus total variable cost.
Labor supply	The number of workers available to an economy. The principal determinants of labor supply are population, real wages, and social traditions.
Total cost	The sum of fixed cost and variable cost is referred to as total cost.
Margin	A deposit by a buyer in stocks with a seller or a stockbroker, as security to cover fluctuations in the market in reference to stocks that the buyer has purchased but for which he has not paid is a margin. Commodities are also traded on margin.
Price variance	The difference between the actual price and the budgeted price multiplied by the actual quantity of input. Also called input-price variance or rate variance.

Chapter 8. Planning and Budgeting

Chapter 8. Planning and Budgeting

Cost overrun	Cost overrun is defined as excess of actual cost over budget. Cost overrun is typically calculated in one of two ways. Either as a percentage, namely actual cost minus budgeted cost, in percent of budgeted cost. Or as a ratio, viz. actual cost divided by budgeted cost.
Usage variance	Usage variance refers to efficiency variance. It is the difference between the budgeted quantity of materials and the actual quantity used. Variance analysis seeks to isolate dollar variances due to usage (using more or less of the correct material) from substitution.
Purchasing	Purchasing refers to the function in a firm that searches for quality material resources, finds the best suppliers, and negotiates the best price for goods and services.
Vendor	A person who sells property to a vendee is a vendor. The words vendor and vendee are more commonly applied to the seller and purchaser of real estate, and the words seller and buyer are more commonly applied to the seller and purchaser of personal property.
Marginal cost	Marginal cost refers to the increase in cost that accompanies a unit increase in output; the partial derivative of the cost function with respect to output.
Aid	Assistance provided by countries and by international institutions such as the World Bank to developing countries in the form of monetary grants, loans at low interest rates, in kind, or a combination of these is called aid. Aid can also refer to assistance of any type rendered to benefit some group or individual.
Cash inflow	Cash coming into the company as the result of a previous investment is a cash inflow.
Liquidity	Liquidity refers to the capacity to turn assets into cash, or the amount of assets in a portfolio that have that capacity.
Peak	Peak refers to the point in the business cycle when an economic expansion reaches its highest point before turning down. Contrasts with trough.
Deficit	The deficit is the amount by which expenditure exceed revenue.
Balance	In banking and accountancy, the outstanding balance is the amount of money owned, (or due), that remains in a deposit account (or a loan account) at a given date, after all past remittances, payments and withdrawal have been accounted for. It can be positive (then, in the balance sheet of a firm, it is an asset) or negative (a liability).
Fixed asset	Fixed asset, also known as property, plant, and equipment (PP&E), is a term used in accountancy for assets and property which cannot easily be converted into cash. This can be compared with current assets such as cash or bank accounts, which are described as liquid assets. In most cases, only tangible assets are referred to as fixed.
Acquisition	A company's purchase of the property and obligations of another company is an acquisition.
Dividend	Amount of corporate profits paid out for each share of stock is referred to as dividend.
Security	Security refers to a claim on the borrower future income that is sold by the borrower to the lender. A security is a type of transferable interest representing financial value.
Marketable securities	Marketable securities refer to securities that are readily traded in the secondary securities market.
Credit	Credit refers to a recording as positive in the balance of payments, any transaction that gives rise to a payment into the country, such as an export, the sale of an asset, or borrowing from abroad.
Foundation	A Foundation is a type of philanthropic organization set up by either individuals or institutions as a legal entity (either as a corporation or trust) with the purpose of distributing grants to support causes in line with the goals of the foundation.
Budget line	Given an allocation of two goods, the budget line through that allocation is the set of all

Chapter 8. Planning and Budgeting

Chapter 8. Planning and Budgeting

	other allocations of the two goods that someone in a market could arrive at by selling one of the goods for the other.
Administration	Administration refers to the management and direction of the affairs of governments and institutions; a collective term for all policymaking officials of a government; the execution and implementation of public policy.
Financial institution	A financial institution acts as an agent that provides financial services for its clients. Financial institutions generally fall under financial regulation from a government authority.
Journal	Book of original entry, in which transactions are recorded in a general ledger system, is referred to as a journal.
Financial management	The job of managing a firm's resources so it can meet its goals and objectives is called financial management.
Strategic management	A philosophy of management that links strategic planning with dayto-day decision making. Strategic management seeks a fit between an organization's external and internal environments.
Capital planning	Capital planning is an accounting process whereby a financial analyst can determine the economic value of business projects/ventures and allocate capital to those endeavors which present the greatest calculated return on investment.
Cost accounting	Cost accounting measures and reports financial and nonfinancial information relating to the cost of acquiring or consuming resources in an organization. It provides information for both management accounting and financial accounting.
Strategic planning	The process of determining the major goals of the organization and the policies and strategies for obtaining and using resources to achieve those goals is called strategic planning.

Chapter 8. Planning and Budgeting

Chapter 9. Time Value Analysis

Future value	Future value measures what money is worth at a specified time in the future assuming a certain interest rate. This is used in time value of money calculations.
Cash flow	In finance, cash flow refers to the amounts of cash being received and spent by a business during a defined period of time, sometimes tied to a specific project. Most of the time they are being used to determine gaps in the liquid position of a company.
Annuities	Financial contracts under which a customer pays an annual premium in exchange for a future stream of annual payments beginning at a set age, say 65, and ending when the person dies are annuities.
Annuity	A contract to make regular payments to a person for life or for a fixed period is an annuity.
Interest rate	The rate of return on bonds, loans, or deposits. When one speaks of 'the' interest rate, it is usually in a model where there is only one.
Interest	In finance and economics, interest is the price paid by a borrower for the use of a lender's money. In other words, interest is the amount of paid to "rent" money for a period of time.
Opportunity cost	The cost of something in terms of opportunity foregone. The opportunity cost to a country of producing a unit more of a good, such as for export or to replace an import, is the quantity of some other good that could have been produced instead.
Cost principle	A principle that holds that it is unethical to charge a higher price for a commodity than the cost of purchasing, producing or acquiring, and bringing it to market is the cost principle.
Investment	Investment refers to spending for the production and accumulation of capital and additions to inventories. In a financial sense, buying an asset with the expectation of making a return.
Ambulatory surgery	Surgery done in the doctor's office or at a surgical center, and not requiring an overnight stay. Ambulatory surgery is general planned ahead of time. Maybe referred to as one-day, in-and-out, or outpatient surgery.
Stock	In financial terminology, stock is the capital raized by a corporation, through the issuance and sale of shares.
Asset	An item of property, such as land, capital, money, a share in ownership, or a claim on others for future payment, such as a bond or a bank deposit is an asset.
Bond	Bond refers to a debt instrument, issued by a borrower and promising a specified stream of payments to the purchaser, usually regular interest payments plus a final repayment of principal.
Timing differences	The difference between the time a transaction occurs and the time the cash related to the transaction is exchanged is referred to as timing differences.
Valuation	In finance, valuation is the process of estimating the market value of a financial asset or liability. They can be done on assets (for example, investments in marketable securities such as stocks, options, business enterprises, or intangible assets such as patents and trademarks) or on liabilities (e.g., Bonds issued by a company).
Value analysis	Value analysis refers to a systematic appraisal of the design, quality, and performance of a product to reduce purchasing costs.
Points	Loan origination fees that may be deductible as interest by a buyer of property. A seller of property who pays points reduces the selling price by the amount of the points paid for the buyer.
Financial management	The job of managing a firm's resources so it can meet its goals and objectives is called financial management.
Management	Management characterizes the process of leading and directing all or part of an organization,

Chapter 9. Time Value Analysis

Chapter 9. Time Value Analysis

	often a business, through the deployment and manipulation of resources. Early twentieth-century management writer Mary Parker Follett defined management as "the art of getting things done through people."
Analyst	Analyst refers to a person or tool with a primary function of information analysis, generally with a more limited, practical and short term set of goals than a researcher.
Present value	The value today of a stream of payments and/or receipts over time in the future and/or the past, converted to the present using an interest rate. If X t is the amount in period t and r the interest rate, then present value at time t=0 is V = ?T /t.
Balance	In banking and accountancy, the outstanding balance is the amount of money owned, (or due), that remains in a deposit account (or a loan account) at a given date, after all past remittances, payments and withdrawal have been accounted for. It can be positive (then, in the balance sheet of a firm, it is an asset) or negative (a liability).
Users	Users refer to people in the organization who actually use the product or service purchased by the buying center.
Argument	The discussion by counsel for the respective parties of their contentions on the law and the facts of the case being tried in order to aid the jury in arriving at a correct and just conclusion is called argument.
Capital budgeting	Capital budgeting is the planning process used to determine a firm's long term investments such as new machinery, replacement machinery, new plants, new products, and research and development projects.
Bond valuation	Bond valuation is the process of determining the fair price of a bond. As with any security, the fair value of a bond is the present value of the stream of cash flows it is expected to generate.
Capital	Capital generally refers to financial wealth, especially that used to start or maintain a business. In classical economics, capital is one of four factors of production, the others being land and labor and entrepreneurship.
Lease	A contract for the possession and use of land or other property, including goods, on one side, and a recompense of rent or other income on the other is the lease.
Mutual fund	A mutual fund is a form of collective investment that pools money from many investors and invests the money in stocks, bonds, short-term money market instruments, and/or other securities. In a mutual fund, the fund manager trades the fund's underlying securities, realizing capital gains or loss, and collects the dividend or interest income.
Fund	Independent accounting entity with a self-balancing set of accounts segregated for the purposes of carrying on specific activities is referred to as a fund.
Security	Security refers to a claim on the borrower future income that is sold by the borrower to the lender. A security is a type of transferable interest representing financial value.
Broker	In commerce, a broker is a party that mediates between a buyer and a seller. A broker who also acts as a seller or as a buyer becomes a principal party to the deal.
Certificate of deposit	An acknowledgment by a bank of the receipt of money with an engagement to pay it back is referred to as certificate of deposit.
Fair value	Fair value is a concept used in finance and economics, defined as a rational and unbiased estimate of the potential market price of a good, service, or asset.
Debt security	Type of security acquired by loaning assets is called a debt security.
Principal	In agency law, one under whose direction an agent acts and for whose benefit that agent acts

Chapter 9. Time Value Analysis

Chapter 9. Time Value Analysis

	is a principal.
Maturity	Maturity refers to the final payment date of a loan or other financial instrument, after which point no further interest or principal need be paid.
Time value of money	Time value of money is the concept that the value of money varies depending on the timing of the cash flows, given any interest rate greater than zero.
Value of money	Value of money refers to the quantity of goods and services for which a unit of money can be exchanged; the purchasing power of a unit of money; the reciprocal of the price level.
Discount rate	Discount rate refers to the rate, per year, at which future values are diminished to make them comparable to values in the present. Can be either subjective or objective.
Discount	The difference between the face value of a bond and its selling price, when a bond is sold for less than its face value it's referred to as a discount.
Acquisition	A company's purchase of the property and obligations of another company is an acquisition.
Cost of capital	Cost of capital refers to the percentage cost of funds used for acquiring resources for an organization, typically a weighted average of the firms cost of equity and cost of debt.
Expected return	Expected return refers to the return on an asset expected over the next period.
Rate of return	A rate of return is a comparison of the money earned (or lost) on an investment to the amount of money invested.
Enterprise	Enterprise refers to another name for a business organization. Other similar terms are business firm, sometimes simply business, sometimes simply firm, as well as company, and entity.
Expected rate of return	Expected rate of return refers to the increase in profit a firm anticipates it will obtain by purchasing capital ; expressed as a percentage of the total cost of the investment activity.
Contribution	In business organization law, the cash or property contributed to a business by its owners is referred to as contribution.
Profit	Profit refers to the return to the resource entrepreneurial ability; total revenue minus total cost.
Future value of an annuity	The sum of the future value of a series of consecutive equal payments is referred to as future value of an annuity.
Present value of an annuity	The sum of the present value of a series of consecutive equal payments is called present value of an annuity.
Perpetuity	A perpetuity is an annuity in which the periodic payments begin on a fixed date and continue indefinitely. Fixed coupon payments on permanently invested (irredeemable) sums of money are prime examples of perpetuities. Scholarships paid perpetually from an endowment fit the definition of perpetuity.
Government bond	A government bond is a bond issued by a national government denominated in the country's own currency. Bonds issued by national governments in foreign currencies are normally referred to as sovereign bonds.
Net present value	Net present value is a standard method in finance of capital budgeting – the planning of long-term investments. Using this method a potential investment project should be undertaken if the present value of all cash inflows minus the present value of all cash outflows (which equals the net present value) is greater than zero.
Cash inflow	Cash coming into the company as the result of a previous investment is a cash inflow.
Trial	An examination before a competent tribunal, according to the law of the land, of the facts or

Chapter 9. Time Value Analysis

Chapter 9. Time Value Analysis

	law put in issue in a cause, for the purpose of determining such issue is a trial. When the court hears and determines any issue of fact or law for the purpose of determining the rights of the parties, it may be considered a trial.
Internal rate of return	Internal rate of return refers to a discounted cash flow method for evaluating capital budgeting projects. The internal rate of return is a discount rate that makes the present value of the cash inflows equal to the present value of the cash outflows.
Compounded semiannually	A compounding period of every six months is called compounded semiannually.
Economy	The income, expenditures, and resources that affect the cost of running a business and household are called an economy.
Effective interest rate	Yield rate of bonds, which is usually equal to the market rate of interest on the day the bonds are sold is the effective interest rate.
Stated interest rate	Rate of interest specified in the bond contract that will be paid at specified intervals over the life of the bond is the stated interest rate.
Mortgage	Mortgage refers to a note payable issued for property, such as a house, usually repaid in equal installments consisting of part principle and part interest, over a specified period.
Amortize	To provide for the payment of a debt by creating a sinking fund or paying in installments is to amortize.
Lender	Suppliers and financial institutions that lend money to companies is referred to as a lender.
Amortization schedule	An amortization schedule is a table detailing each periodic payment on a loan (typically a mortgage), as generated by an amortization calculator. They are calculated so that each periodic payment for the entirety of the loan is equal, making the repayment process somewhat simpler under amortization than with other models.
Amortization	Systematic and rational allocation of the acquisition cost of an intangible asset over its useful life is referred to as amortization.
Contract	A contract is a "promise" or an "agreement" that is enforced or recognized by the law. In the civil law, a contract is considered to be part of the general law of obligations.
Net income	Net income is equal to the income that a firm has after subtracting costs and expenses from the total revenue. Expenses will typically include tax expense.
Refunding	The process of retiring an old bond issue before maturity and replacing it with a new issue is refunding. Refunding will occur when interest rates have fallen and new bonds may be sold at lower interest rates.
Term loan	Term loan refers to an intermediate-length loan, in which credit is generally extended from one to seven years. The loan is usually repaid in monthly or quarterly installments over its life, rather than with one single payment.
Corporation	A legal entity chartered by a state or the Federal government that is distinct and separate from the individuals who own it is a corporation. This separation gives the corporation unique powers which other legal entities lack.
Dividend	Amount of corporate profits paid out for each share of stock is referred to as dividend.
Consumption	In Keynesian economics consumption refers to personal consumption expenditure, i.e., the purchase of currently produced goods and services out of income, out of savings (net worth), or from borrowed funds. It refers to that part of disposable income that does not go to saving.
Variable	A variable is something measured by a number; it is used to analyze what happens to other

Chapter 9. Time Value Analysis

Chapter 9. Time Value Analysis

	things when the size of that number changes.
Diversification	Investing in a collection of assets whose returns do not always move together, with the result that overall risk is lower than for individual assets is referred to as diversification.
Firm	An organization that employs resources to produce a good or service for profit and owns and operates one or more plants is referred to as a firm.
Financial institution	A financial institution acts as an agent that provides financial services for its clients. Financial institutions generally fall under financial regulation from a government authority.
Yield	The interest rate that equates a future value or an annuity to a given present value is a yield.
Annual percentage rate	Annual percentage rate refers to a measure of the effective rate on a loan. One uses the actuarial method of compound interest when calculating the annual percentage rate.
Credit	Credit refers to a recording as positive in the balance of payments, any transaction that gives rise to a payment into the country, such as an export, the sale of an asset, or borrowing from abroad.

Chapter 9. Time Value Analysis

Chapter 10. Financial Risk and Required Return

Portfolio	In finance, a portfolio is a collection of investments held by an institution or a private individual. Holding but not always a portfolio is part of an investment and risk-limiting strategy called diversification. By owning several assets, certain types of risk (in particular specific risk) can be reduced.
Market risk	Market risk is the risk that the value of an investment will decrease due to moves in market factors.
Market	A market is, as defined in economics, a social arrangement that allows buyers and sellers to discover information and carry out a voluntary exchange of goods or services.
Rate of return	A rate of return is a comparison of the money earned (or lost) on an investment to the amount of money invested.
Required rate of return	Required rate of return refers to the rate of return that investors demand from an investment to compensate them for the amount of risk involved.
Financial management	The job of managing a firm's resources so it can meet its goals and objectives is called financial management.
Financial risk	The risk related to the inability of the firm to meet its debt obligations as they come due is called financial risk.
Management	Management characterizes the process of leading and directing all or part of an organization, often a business, through the deployment and manipulation of resources. Early twentieth-century management writer Mary Parker Follett defined management as "the art of getting things done through people."
Appreciation	Appreciation refers to a rise in the value of a country's currency on the exchange market, relative either to a particular other currency or to a weighted average of other currencies. The currency is said to appreciate. Opposite of 'depreciation.' Appreciation can also refer to the increase in value of any asset.
Gain	In finance, gain is a profit or an increase in value of an investment such as a stock or bond. Gain is calculated by fair market value or the proceeds from the sale of the investment minus the sum of the purchase price and all costs associated with it.
Service	Service refers to a "non tangible product" that is not embodied in a physical good and that typically effects some change in another product, person, or institution. Contrasts with good.
Context	The effect of the background under which a message often takes on more and richer meaning is a context. Context is especially important in cross-cultural interactions because some cultures are said to be high context or low context.
Capital	Capital generally refers to financial wealth, especially that used to start or maintain a business. In classical economics, capital is one of four factors of production, the others being land and labor and entrepreneurship.
Supply	Supply is the aggregate amount of any material good that can be called into being at a certain price point; it comprises one half of the equation of supply and demand. In classical economic theory, a curve representing supply is one of the factors that produce price.
Investment	Investment refers to spending for the production and accumulation of capital and additions to inventories. In a financial sense, buying an asset with the expectation of making a return.
Interest	In finance and economics, interest is the price paid by a borrower for the use of a lender's money. In other words, interest is the amount of paid to "rent" money for a period of time.
Residual	Residual payments can refer to an ongoing stream of payments in respect of the completion of past achievements.

Go to **Cram101.com** for the Practice Tests for this Chapter.

Chapter 10. Financial Risk and Required Return

Chapter 10. Financial Risk and Required Return

Stockholder	A stockholder is an individual or company (including a corporation) that legally owns one or more shares of stock in a joined stock company. The shareholders are the owners of a corporation. Companies listed at the stock market strive to enhance shareholder value.
Cash flow	In finance, cash flow refers to the amounts of cash being received and spent by a business during a defined period of time, sometimes tied to a specific project. Most of the time they are being used to determine gaps in the liquid position of a company.
Equity	Equity is the name given to the set of legal principles, in countries following the English common law tradition, which supplement strict rules of law where their application would operate harshly, so as to achieve what is sometimes referred to as "natural justice."
Asset	An item of property, such as land, capital, money, a share in ownership, or a claim on others for future payment, such as a bond or a bank deposit is an asset.
Stock	In financial terminology, stock is the capital raized by a corporation, through the issuance and sale of shares.
Bond	Bond refers to a debt instrument, issued by a borrower and promising a specified stream of payments to the purchaser, usually regular interest payments plus a final repayment of principal.
Contract	A contract is a "promise" or an "agreement" that is enforced or recognized by the law. In the civil law, a contract is considered to be part of the general law of obligations.
Maturity	Maturity refers to the final payment date of a loan or other financial instrument, after which point no further interest or principal need be paid.
Partnership	In the common law, a partnership is a type of business entity in which partners share with each other the profits or losses of the business undertaking in which they have all invested.
Interest rate	The rate of return on bonds, loans, or deposits. When one speaks of 'the' interest rate, it is usually in a model where there is only one.
Future value	Future value measures what money is worth at a specified time in the future assuming a certain interest rate. This is used in time value of money calculations.
Dividend	Amount of corporate profits paid out for each share of stock is referred to as dividend.
Cash inflow	Cash coming into the company as the result of a previous investment is a cash inflow.
Discount	The difference between the face value of a bond and its selling price, when a bond is sold for less than its face value it's referred to as a discount.
Weighted average	The weighted average unit cost of the goods available for sale for both cost of goods sold and ending inventory.
Distribution	Distribution in economics, the manner in which total output and income is distributed among individuals or factors.
Expected rate of return	Expected rate of return refers to the increase in profit a firm anticipates it will obtain by purchasing capital ; expressed as a percentage of the total cost of the investment activity.
Expected return	Expected return refers to the return on an asset expected over the next period.
Standard deviation	A measure of the spread or dispersion of a series of numbers around the expected value is the standard deviation. The standard deviation tells us how well the expected value represents a series of values.
Expected value	A representative value from a probability distribution arrived at by multiplying each outcome by the associated probability and summing up the values is called the expected value.
Variance	Variance refers to a measure of how much an economic or statistical variable varies across

Chapter 10. Financial Risk and Required Return

Chapter 10. Financial Risk and Required Return

	values or observations. Its calculation is the same as that of the covariance, being the covariance of the variable with itself.
Return on investment	Return on investment refers to the return a businessperson gets on the money he and other owners invest in the firm; for example, a business that earned $100 on a $1,000 investment would have a ROI of 10 percent: 100 divided by 1000.
Security	Security refers to a claim on the borrower future income that is sold by the borrower to the lender. A security is a type of transferable interest representing financial value.
Investment portfolio	An investment portfolio is an aggregate of investments, such as stocks, bonds, real estate, arts or even fine wines. What distinguishes an investment portfolio from net worth is that some asset classes are not considered investments.
Correlation	A correlation is the measure of the extent to which two economic or statistical variables move together, normalized so that its values range from -1 to +1. It is defined as the covariance of the two variables divided by the square root of the product of their variances.
Variable	A variable is something measured by a number; it is used to analyze what happens to other things when the size of that number changes.
Positively correlated	Positively correlated refers to values or amounts of two items that move in the same direction. In accounting and finance, the amount of risk and the amount of return on an investment move in the same direction.
Forming	The first stage of team development, where the team is formed and the objectives for the team are set is referred to as forming.
Industry	A group of firms that produce identical or similar products is an industry. It is also used specifically to refer to an area of economic production focused on manufacturing which involves large amounts of capital investment before any profit can be realized, also called "heavy industry".
Holding	The holding is a court's determination of a matter of law based on the issue presented in the particular case. In other words: under this law, with these facts, this result.
Mutual fund	A mutual fund is a form of collective investment that pools money from many investors and invests the money in stocks, bonds, short-term money market instruments, and/or other securities. In a mutual fund, the fund manager trades the fund's underlying securities, realizing capital gains or loss, and collects the dividend or interest income.
Fund	Independent accounting entity with a self-balancing set of accounts segregated for the purposes of carrying on specific activities is referred to as a fund.
Stock exchange	A stock exchange is a corporation or mutual organization which provides facilities for stock brokers and traders, to trade company stocks and other securities.
Common stock	Common stock refers to the basic, normal, voting stock issued by a corporation; called residual equity because it ranks after preferred stock for dividend and liquidation distributions.
Exchange	The trade of things of value between buyer and seller so that each is better off after the trade is called the exchange.
Recession	A significant decline in economic activity. In the U.S., recession is approximately defined as two successive quarters of falling GDP, as judged by NBER.
Economy	The income, expenditures, and resources that affect the cost of running a business and household are called an economy.
Diversification	Investing in a collection of assets whose returns do not always move together, with the

Go to **Cram101.com** for the Practice Tests for this Chapter.

Chapter 10. Financial Risk and Required Return

Chapter 10. Financial Risk and Required Return

	result that overall risk is lower than for individual assets is referred to as diversification.
Strike	The withholding of labor services by an organized group of workers is referred to as a strike.
Firm	An organization that employs resources to produce a good or service for profit and owns and operates one or more plants is referred to as a firm.
Trend	Trend refers to the long-term movement of an economic variable, such as its average rate of increase or decrease over enough years to encompass several business cycles.
Inflation	An increase in the overall price level of an economy, usually as measured by the CPI or by the implicit price deflator is called inflation.
Diversified portfolio	Diversified portfolio refers to a portfolio that includes a variety of assets whose prices are not likely all to change together. In international economics, this usually means holding assets denominated in different currencies.
Contribution	In business organization law, the cash or property contributed to a business by its owners is referred to as contribution.
Beta coefficient	The Beta coefficient (sensitivity of the asset returns to market returns, relative volatility), is a key parameter in the Capital asset pricing model. It can also be defined as the risk of the stock to a diversified portfolio.
Volatility	Volatility refers to the extent to which an economic variable, such as a price or an exchange rate, moves up and down over time.
Regression line	A line fit to a set of data points using least-squares regression is referred to as a regression line.
Slope	The slope of a line in the plane containing the x and y axes is generally represented by the letter m, and is defined as the change in the y coordinate divided by the corresponding change in the x coordinate, between two distinct points on the line.
Economic forces	Forces that affect the availability, production, and distribution of a society's resources among competing users are referred to as economic forces.
Points	Loan origination fees that may be deductible as interest by a buyer of property. A seller of property who pays points reduces the selling price by the amount of the points paid for the buyer.
Above the line	Above the line is an advertising technique using mass media to promote brands. This type of communication is conventional in nature and is considered impersonal to customers.
Below the line	Below the line is an advertising technique. It uses less conventional methods than the usual specific channels of advertising to promote products, services, etc. than ATL (Above the line) strategy.
Closing	The finalization of a real estate sales transaction that passes title to the property from the seller to the buyer is referred to as a closing. Closing is a sales term which refers to the process of making a sale. It refers to reaching the final step, which may be an exchange of money or acquiring a signature.
Equity capital	Equity capital refers to money raized from within the firm or through the sale of ownership in the firm.
Opportunity cost	The cost of something in terms of opportunity foregone. The opportunity cost to a country of producing a unit more of a good, such as for export or to replace an import, is the quantity of some other good that could have been produced instead.

Chapter 10. Financial Risk and Required Return

Chapter 10. Financial Risk and Required Return

Consideration	Consideration in contract law, a basic requirement for an enforceable agreement under traditional contract principles, defined in this text as legal value, bargained for and given in exchange for an act or promise. In corporation law, cash or property contributed to a corporation in exchange for shares, or a promise to contribute such cash or property.
Shareholder wealth maximization	Shareholder wealth maximization refers to maximizing the wealth of the firm's shareholders through achieving the highest possible value for the firm in the marketplace. It is the overriding objective of the firm and should influence all decisions.
Shareholder	A shareholder is an individual or company (including a corporation) that legally owns one or more shares of stock in a joined stock company.
Equity investment	Equity investment generally refers to the buying and holding of shares of stock on a stock market by individuals and funds in anticipation of income from dividends and capital gain as the value of the stock rises.
Mission statement	Mission statement refers to an outline of the fundamental purposes of an organization.
Capital asset pricing model	The capital asset pricing model is used in finance to determine a theoretically appropriate required rate of return (and thus the price if expected cash flows can be estimated) of an asset, if that asset is to be added to an already well-diversified portfolio, given that asset's non-diversifiable risk.
Capital asset	In accounting, a capital asset is an asset that is recorded as property that creates more property, e.g. a factory that creates shoes, or a forest that yields a quantity of wood.
Market risk premium	Market risk premium refers to a premium over and above the risk-free rate. It is represented by the difference between the market return and the risk-free rate, and it may be multiplied by the beta coefficient to determine the additional risk-adjusted return on a security.
Risk premium	In finance, the risk premium can be the expected rate of return above the risk-free interest rate.
Premium	Premium refers to the fee charged by an insurance company for an insurance policy. The rate of losses must be relatively predictable: In order to set the premium (prices) insurers must be able to estimate them accurately.
Risk aversion	Risk aversion is the reluctance of a person to accept a bargain with an uncertain payoff rather than another bargain with a more certain but possibly lower expected payoff.
Security market line	A line or equation that depicts the risk-related return of a security based on a risk-free rate plus a market premium related to the beta coefficient of the security is referred to as the security market line.
Corporation	A legal entity chartered by a state or the Federal government that is distinct and separate from the individuals who own it is a corporation. This separation gives the corporation unique powers which other legal entities lack.
Analyst	Analyst refers to a person or tool with a primary function of information analysis, generally with a more limited, practical and short term set of goals than a researcher.

Chapter 10. Financial Risk and Required Return

Chapter 11. Long-Term Debt Financing

Instrument	Instrument refers to an economic variable that is controlled by policy makers and can be used to influence other variables, called targets. Examples are monetary and fiscal policies used to achieve external and internal balance.
Interest rate	The rate of return on bonds, loans, or deposits. When one speaks of 'the' interest rate, it is usually in a model where there is only one.
Interest	In finance and economics, interest is the price paid by a borrower for the use of a lender's money. In other words, interest is the amount of paid to "rent" money for a period of time.
Asset	An item of property, such as land, capital, money, a share in ownership, or a claim on others for future payment, such as a bond or a bank deposit is an asset.
Capital	Capital generally refers to financial wealth, especially that used to start or maintain a business. In classical economics, capital is one of four factors of production, the others being land and labor and entrepreneurship.
Equity	Equity is the name given to the set of legal principles, in countries following the English common law tradition, which supplement strict rules of law where their application would operate harshly, so as to achieve what is sometimes referred to as "natural justice."
Retained earnings	Cumulative earnings of a company that are not distributed to the owners and are reinvested in the business are called retained earnings.
Equity capital	Equity capital refers to money raized from within the firm or through the sale of ownership in the firm.
Contribution	In business organization law, the cash or property contributed to a business by its owners is referred to as contribution.
Stockholder	A stockholder is an individual or company (including a corporation) that legally owns one or more shares of stock in a joined stock company. The shareholders are the owners of a corporation. Companies listed at the stock market strive to enhance shareholder value.
Corporation	A legal entity chartered by a state or the Federal government that is distinct and separate from the individuals who own it is a corporation. This separation gives the corporation unique powers which other legal entities lack.
Grant	Grant refers to an intergovernmental transfer of funds . Since the New Deal, state and local governments have become increasingly dependent upon federal grants for an almost infinite variety of programs.
Fund	Independent accounting entity with a self-balancing set of accounts segregated for the purposes of carrying on specific activities is referred to as a fund.
Fixed cost	The cost that a firm bears if it does not produce at all and that is independent of its output. The presence of a fixed cost tends to imply increasing returns to scale. Contrasts with variable cost.
Equity financing	Financing that consists of funds that are invested in exchange for ownership in the company is called equity financing.
Debt financing	Obtaining financing by borrowing money is debt financing.
Creditor	A person to whom a debt or legal obligation is owed, and who has the right to enforce payment of that debt or obligation is referred to as creditor.
Debt capital	Debt capital refers to funds raized through various forms of borrowing to finance a company that must be repaid.
Firm	An organization that employs resources to produce a good or service for profit and owns and operates one or more plants is referred to as a firm.

Chapter 11. Long-Term Debt Financing

Chapter 11. Long-Term Debt Financing

Consumption	In Keynesian economics consumption refers to personal consumption expenditure, i.e., the purchase of currently produced goods and services out of income, out of savings (net worth), or from borrowed funds. It refers to that part of disposable income that does not go to saving.
Investment	Investment refers to spending for the production and accumulation of capital and additions to inventories. In a financial sense, buying an asset with the expectation of making a return.
Preference	The act of a debtor in paying or securing one or more of his creditors in a manner more favorable to them than to other creditors or to the exclusion of such other creditors is a preference. In the absence of statute, a preference is perfectly good, but to be legal it must be bona fide, and not a mere subterfuge of the debtor to secure a future benefit to himself or to prevent the application of his property to his debts.
Inflation	An increase in the overall price level of an economy, usually as measured by the CPI or by the implicit price deflator is called inflation.
Supply	Supply is the aggregate amount of any material good that can be called into being at a certain price point; it comprises one half of the equation of supply and demand. In classical economic theory, a curve representing supply is one of the factors that produce price.
Entrepreneur	The owner/operator. The person who organizes, manages, and assumes the risks of a firm, taking a new idea or a new product and turning it into a successful business is an entrepreneur.
Lender	Suppliers and financial institutions that lend money to companies is referred to as a lender.
Capital formation	Capital formation is synonymous with investment. It refers to the process of building up the capital stock.
Economy	The income, expenditures, and resources that affect the cost of running a business and household are called an economy.
Value of money	Value of money refers to the quantity of goods and services for which a unit of money can be exchanged; the purchasing power of a unit of money; the reciprocal of the price level.
Purchasing power	The amount of goods that money will buy, usually measured by the CPI is referred to as purchasing power.
Purchasing	Purchasing refers to the function in a firm that searches for quality material resources, finds the best suppliers, and negotiates the best price for goods and services.
Mortgage	Mortgage refers to a note payable issued for property, such as a house, usually repaid in equal installments consisting of part principle and part interest, over a specified period.
Principal	In agency law, one under whose direction an agent acts and for whose benefit that agent acts is a principal.
Term loan	Term loan refers to an intermediate-length loan, in which credit is generally extended from one to seven years. The loan is usually repaid in monthly or quarterly installments over its life, rather than with one single payment.
Contract	A contract is a "promise" or an "agreement" that is enforced or recognized by the law. In the civil law, a contract is considered to be part of the general law of obligations.
Investment banker	Investment banker refers to a financial organization that specializes in selling primary offerings of securities. Investment bankers can also perform other financial functions, such as advising clients, negotiating mergers and takeovers, and selling secondary offerings.
Financial institution	A financial institution acts as an agent that provides financial services for its clients. Financial institutions generally fall under financial regulation from a government authority.

Go to Cram101.com for the Practice Tests for this Chapter.

Chapter 11. Long-Term Debt Financing

Chapter 11. Long-Term Debt Financing

Commercial bank	A firm that engages in the business of banking is a commercial bank.
Pension fund	Amounts of money put aside by corporations, nonprofit organizations, or unions to cover part of the financial needs of members when they retire is a pension fund.
Mutual fund	A mutual fund is a form of collective investment that pools money from many investors and invests the money in stocks, bonds, short-term money market instruments, and/or other securities. In a mutual fund, the fund manager trades the fund's underlying securities, realizing capital gains or loss, and collects the dividend or interest income.
Insurance	Insurance refers to a system by which individuals can reduce their exposure to risk of large losses by spreading the risks among a large number of persons.
Pension	A pension is a steady income given to a person (usually after retirement). Pensions are typically payments made in the form of a guaranteed annuity to a retired or disabled employee.
Maturity	Maturity refers to the final payment date of a loan or other financial instrument, after which point no further interest or principal need be paid.
Variable	A variable is something measured by a number; it is used to analyze what happens to other things when the size of that number changes.
Bond	Bond refers to a debt instrument, issued by a borrower and promising a specified stream of payments to the purchaser, usually regular interest payments plus a final repayment of principal.
Prime rate	The rate that a bank charges its most creditworthy customers is referred to as the prime rate.
Points	Loan origination fees that may be deductible as interest by a buyer of property. A seller of property who pays points reduces the selling price by the amount of the points paid for the buyer.
Balance	In banking and accountancy, the outstanding balance is the amount of money owned, (or due), that remains in a deposit account (or a loan account) at a given date, after all past remittances, payments and withdrawal have been accounted for. It can be positive (then, in the balance sheet of a firm, it is an asset) or negative (a liability).
Holder	A person in possession of a document of title or an instrument payable or indorsed to him, his order, or to bearer is a holder.
Federal government	Federal government refers to the government of the United States, as distinct from the state and local governments.
Corporate bond	A Corporate bond is a bond issued by a corporation, as the name suggests. The term is usually applied to longer term debt instruments, generally with a maturity date falling at least 12 months after their issue date (the term "commercial paper" being sometimes used for instruments with a shorter maturity).
Municipal bond	In the United States, a municipal bond is a bond issued by a state, city or other local government, or their agencies. Potential issuers of these include cities, counties, redevelopment agencies, school districts, publicly owned airports and seaports, and any other governmental entity (or group of governments) below the state level. They are guaranteed by a local government, a subdivision thereof, or a group of local governments, and are assessed for risk and rated accordingly.
Fixed interest rate	Interest rate that does not change over the life of the loan is called the fixed interest rate. A rate that does not fluctuate with general market conditions.
Interest payment	The payment to holders of bonds payable, calculated by multiplying the stated rate on the

Chapter 11. Long-Term Debt Financing

Chapter 11. Long-Term Debt Financing

	face of the bond by the par, or face, value of the bond. If bonds are issued at a discount or premium, the interest payment does not equal the interest expense.
Fixed interest	A fixed interest rate loan is a loan where the interest rate doesn't fluctuate over the life of the loan. This allows the borrower to accurately predict their future payments. When the prevailing interest rate is very low, a fixed rate loan will be slightly higher than variable rate loans because the lender is taking a risk they he could get a higher interest rate by loaning money later.
Mortgage bond	Type of secured bond that conditionally transfers title of a designated piece of property to the bondholder until the bond is paid is referred to as mortgage bond.
Security	Security refers to a claim on the borrower future income that is sold by the borrower to the lender. A security is a type of transferable interest representing financial value.
Issuer	The company that borrows money from investors by issuing bonds is referred to as issuer. They are legally responsible for the obligations of the issue and for reporting financial conditions, material developments and any other operational activities as required by the regulations of their jurisdictions.
Pledge	In law a pledge (also pawn) is a bailment of personal property as a security for some debt or engagement.
Bondholder	The individual or entity that purchases a bond, thus loaning money to the company that issued the bond is the bondholder.
Default	In finance, default occurs when a debtor has not met its legal obligations according to the debt contract, e.g. it has not made a scheduled payment, or violated a covenant (condition) of the debt contract.
Liquidation	Liquidation refers to a process whereby the assets of a business are converted to money. The conversion may be coerced by a legal process to pay off the debt of the business, or to satisfy any other business obligation that the business has not voluntarily satisfied.
Bankruptcy	Bankruptcy is a legally declared inability or impairment of ability of an individual or organization to pay their creditors.
Property	Assets defined in the broadest legal sense. Property includes the unrealized receivables of a cash basis taxpayer, but not services rendered.
Unsecured bond	A bond backed only by the reputation of the issuer is an unsecured bond. A bond not backed by collateral, also called debentures.
Debenture	A debenture is a long-term debt instrument used by governments and large companies to obtain funds. It is similar to a bond except the securitization conditions are different.
Lien	In its most extensive meaning, it is a charge on property for the payment or discharge of a debt or duty is referred to as lien.
Credit	Credit refers to a recording as positive in the balance of payments, any transaction that gives rise to a payment into the country, such as an export, the sale of an asset, or borrowing from abroad.
Collateral	Property that is pledged to the lender to guarantee payment in the event that the borrower is unable to make debt payments is called collateral.
Subordinated debenture	An unsecured bond, in which payment to the holder will occur only after designated senior debenture holders are satisfied is a subordinated debenture.
Authority	Authority in agency law, refers to an agent's ability to affect his principal's legal relations with third parties. Also used to refer to an actor's legal power or ability to do

Go to **Cram101.com** for the Practice Tests for this Chapter.

Chapter 11. Long-Term Debt Financing

Chapter 11. Long-Term Debt Financing

	something. In addition, sometimes used to refer to a statute, case, or other legal source that justifies a particular result.
Municipal securities	Municipal securities refer to securities issued by state and local government units. The income from these securities is exempt from federal income taxes.
Revenue bond	A revenue bond is a special type of municipal bond distinguished by its guarantee of repayment solely from revenues generated by a specified revenue-generating entity associated with the purpose of the bonds.
Revenue	Revenue is a U.S. business term for the amount of money that a company receives from its activities, mostly from sales of products and/or services to customers.
Gain	In finance, gain is a profit or an increase in value of an investment such as a stock or bond. Gain is calculated by fair market value or the proceeds from the sale of the investment minus the sum of the purchase price and all costs associated with it.
Debt service	The payments made by a borrower on their debt, usually including both interest payments and partial repayment of principal, are called debt service.
Service	Service refers to a "non tangible product" that is not embodied in a physical good and that typically effects some change in another product, person, or institution. Contrasts with good.
Yield	The interest rate that equates a future value or an annuity to a given present value is a yield.
Public placement	Public placement refers to the sale of securities to the public through the investment banker-underwriter process. Public placements must be registered with the Securities and Exchange Commission.
Goldman Sachs	Goldman Sachs is widely respected as a financial advisor to some of the most important companies, largest governments, and wealthiest families in the world. It is a primary dealer in the U.S. Treasury securities market. It offers its clients mergers & acquisitions advisory, provides underwriting services, engages in proprietary trading, invests in private equity deals, and also manages the wealth of affluent individuals and families.
Underwriters	Investment banks that guarantee prices on securities to corporations and then sell the securities to the public are underwriters.
Institutional investors	Institutional investors refers to large organizations such as pension funds, mutual funds, insurance companies, and banks that invest their own funds or the funds of others.
Administrative cost	An administrative cost is all executive, organizational, and clerical costs associated with the general management of an organization rather than with manufacturing, marketing, or selling
Private placement	Private placement refers to the sale of securities directly to a financial institution by a corporation. This eliminates the middleman and reduces the cost of issue to the corporation.
Accounting	A system that collects and processes financial information about an organization and reports that information to decision makers is referred to as accounting.
Indenture	A bond contract that specifies the legal provisions of a bond issue is called an indenture.
Cost of debt	The cost of debt is the cost of borrowing money (usually denoted by Kd). It is derived by dividing debt's interest payments on the total market value of the debts.
Restrictive covenant	A restrictive covenant is a legal obligation imposed in a deed by the seller upon the buyer of real estate to do or not to do something.
Covenant	A covenant is a signed written agreement between two or more parties. Also referred to as a

Go to Cram101.com for the Practice Tests for this Chapter.

Chapter 11. Long-Term Debt Financing

Chapter 11. Long-Term Debt Financing

	contract.
Current ratio	The current ratio is a comparison of a firm's current assets to its current liabilities. The current ratio is an indication of a firm's market liquidity and ability to meet short-term debt obligations.
Trustee	An independent party appointed to represent the bondholders is referred to as a trustee.
Call provision	Call provision refers to bonds and some preferred stock, in which a call allows the corporation to retire securities before maturity by forcing the bondholders to sell bonds back to it at a set price. The call provisions are included in the bond indenture.
Call premium	The call premium is the amount over par value an issuer must pay to redeem a callable bond on a call date.
Premium	Premium refers to the fee charged by an insurance company for an insurance policy. The rate of losses must be relatively predictable: In order to set the premium (prices) insurers must be able to estimate them accurately.
Callable bond	A callable bond is a bond that can be redeemed by the issuer prior to its maturity, on certain dates, at a price determined at issuance.
Privilege	Generally, a legal right to engage in conduct that would otherwise result in legal liability is a privilege. Privileges are commonly classified as absolute or conditional. Occasionally, privilege is also used to denote a legal right to refrain from particular behavior.
Interest expense	The cost a business incurs to borrow money. With respect to bonds payable, the interest expense is calculated by multiplying the market rate of interest by the carrying value of the bonds on the date of the payment.
Expense	In accounting, an expense represents an event in which an asset is used up or a liability is incurred. In terms of the accounting equation, expenses reduce owners' equity.
Debt security	Type of security acquired by loaning assets is called a debt security.
Refunding	The process of retiring an old bond issue before maturity and replacing it with a new issue is refunding. Refunding will occur when interest rates have fallen and new bonds may be sold at lower interest rates.
Future interest	Future interest refers to an interest that will come into being at some future time. It is distinguished from a present interest, which already exists. Assume that Dan transfers securities to a newly created trust.
Bond ratings	Bond ratings refers to rating of bonds according to risk by Standard & Poor's and Moody's Investor Service. A bond that is rated A by Moody's has the lowest risk, while a bond with a C rating has the highest risk. Coupon rates are greatly influenced by a corporation's bond rating.
Junk bond	In finance, a junk bond is a bond that is rated below investment grade. These bonds have a higher risk of defaulting, but typically pay high yields in order to make them attractive to investors.
Analyst	Analyst refers to a person or tool with a primary function of information analysis, generally with a more limited, practical and short term set of goals than a researcher.
General Electric	In 1876, Thomas Alva Edison opened a new laboratory in Menlo Park, New Jersey. Out of the laboratory was to come perhaps the most famous invention of all—a successful development of the incandescent electric lamp. By 1890, Edison had organized his various businesses into the Edison General Electric Company.
Subsidiary	A company that is controlled by another company or corporation is a subsidiary.

Go to **Cram101.com** for the Practice Tests for this Chapter.

Chapter 11. Long-Term Debt Financing

Chapter 11. Long-Term Debt Financing

Guaranty	An undertaking by one person to be answerable for the payment of some debt, or the due performance of some contract or duty by another person, who remains liable to pay or perform the same is called guaranty.
Basis point	One one-hundredth of a percentage point is a basis point. Each one percent in interest is equal to 100 basis points.
Capital asset pricing model	The capital asset pricing model is used in finance to determine a theoretically appropriate required rate of return (and thus the price if expected cash flows can be estimated) of an asset, if that asset is to be added to an already well-diversified portfolio, given that asset's non-diversifiable risk.
Rate of return	A rate of return is a comparison of the money earned (or lost) on an investment to the amount of money invested.
Capital asset	In accounting, a capital asset is an asset that is recorded as property that creates more property, e.g. a factory that creates shoes, or a forest that yields a quantity of wood.
Stock	In financial terminology, stock is the capital raized by a corporation, through the issuance and sale of shares.
Inflation premium	Inflation premium refers to a premium to compensate the investor for the eroding effect of inflation on the value of the dollar. The inflation premium ensures that you do not lose the purchasing power of your investment over time.
Inflation rate	The percentage increase in the price level per year is an inflation rate. Alternatively, the inflation rate is the rate of decrease in the purchasing power of money.
Market price	Market price is an economic concept with commonplace familiarity; it is the price that a good or service is offered at, or will fetch, in the marketplace; it is of interest mainly in the study of microeconomics.
Liquidity	Liquidity refers to the capacity to turn assets into cash, or the amount of assets in a portfolio that have that capacity.
Market	A market is, as defined in economics, a social arrangement that allows buyers and sellers to discover information and carry out a voluntary exchange of goods or services.
Treasury security	A treasury security is a government bond issued by the United States Department of the Treasury through the Bureau of the Public Debt. They are the debt financing instruments of the U.S. Federal government, and are often referred to simply as Treasuries.
Default risk	The chance that the issuer of a debt instrument will be unable to make interest payments or pay off the face value when the instrument matures is called default risk.
Bond valuation	Bond valuation is the process of determining the fair price of a bond. As with any security, the fair value of a bond is the present value of the stream of cash flows it is expected to generate.
Risk premium	In finance, the risk premium can be the expected rate of return above the risk-free interest rate.
Market value	Market value refers to the price of an asset agreed on between a willing buyer and a willing seller; the price an asset could demand if it is sold on the open market.
Valuation	In finance, valuation is the process of estimating the market value of a financial asset or liability. They can be done on assets (for example, investments in marketable securities such as stocks, options, business enterprises, or intangible assets such as patents and trademarks) or on liabilities (e.g., Bonds issued by a company).
Deferral	Deferred is any account where the asset or liability is not realized until a future date,

Chapter 11. Long-Term Debt Financing

Chapter 11. Long-Term Debt Financing

	e.g. annuities, charges, taxes, income, etc. The deferred item may be carried, dependent on type of deferral, as either an asset or liability.
Economic forces	Forces that affect the availability, production, and distribution of a society's resources among competing users are referred to as economic forces.
Term structure of interest rates	The relationship among interest rates on bonds with different terms to maturity is referred to as term structure of interest rates.
Wall Street Journal	Dow Jones & Company was founded in 1882 by reporters Charles Dow, Edward Jones and Charles Bergstresser. Jones converted the small Customers' Afternoon Letter into The Wall Street Journal, first published in 1889, and began delivery of the Dow Jones News Service via telegraph. The Journal featured the Jones 'Average', the first of several indexes of stock and bond prices on the New York Stock Exchange.
Journal	Book of original entry, in which transactions are recorded in a general ledger system, is referred to as a journal.
Yield curve	In finance, the yield curve is the relation between the interest rate (or cost of borrowing) and the maturity of the debt for a given borrower in a given currency.
Slope	The slope of a line in the plane containing the x and y axes is generally represented by the letter m, and is defined as the change in the y coordinate divided by the corresponding change in the x coordinate, between two distinct points on the line.
Normal yield curve	Normal yield curve refers to an upward-sloping yield curve. Long-term interest rates are higher than short-term rates.
Policy	Similar to a script in that a policy can be a less than completely rational decision-making method. Involves the use of a pre-existing set of decision steps for any problem that presents itself.
Cash flow	In finance, cash flow refers to the amounts of cash being received and spent by a business during a defined period of time, sometimes tied to a specific project. Most of the time they are being used to determine gaps in the liquid position of a company.
Distribution	Distribution in economics, the manner in which total output and income is distributed among individuals or factors.
Probability distribution	A specification of the probabilities for each possible value of a random variable is called probability distribution.
Required rate of return	Required rate of return refers to the rate of return that investors demand from an investment to compensate them for the amount of risk involved.
Present value	The value today of a stream of payments and/or receipts over time in the future and/or the past, converted to the present using an interest rate. If X_t is the amount in period t and r the interest rate, then present value at time t=0 is $V = ?T /t$.
Frequency	Frequency refers to the speed of the up and down movements of a fluctuating economic variable; that is, the number of times per unit of time that the variable completes a cycle of up and down movement.
Financial assets	Financial assets refer to monetary claims or obligations by one party against another party. Examples are bonds, mortgages, bank loans, and equities.
Par value	The central value of a pegged exchange rate, around which the actual rate is permitted to fluctuate within set bounds is a par value.
Maturity date	The date on which the final payment on a bond is due from the bond issuer to the investor is

Go to **Cram101.com** for the Practice Tests for this Chapter.

Chapter 11. Long-Term Debt Financing

Chapter 11. Long-Term Debt Financing

	a maturity date.
Coupon rate	In bonds, notes or other fixed income securities, the stated percentage rate of interest, usually paid twice a year is the coupon rate.
Coupon	In finance, a coupon is "attached" to a bond, either physically (as with old bonds) or electronically. Each coupon represents a predetermined payment promized to the bond-holder in return for his or her loan of money to the bond-issuer. .
Seasoned issue	A stock issued for sale for which prior issues currently sell in the market is called a seasoned issue.
Discount rate	Discount rate refers to the rate, per year, at which future values are diminished to make them comparable to values in the present. Can be either subjective or objective .
Discount	The difference between the face value of a bond and its selling price, when a bond is sold for less than its face value it's referred to as a discount.
Annuity	A contract to make regular payments to a person for life or for a fixed period is an annuity.
Bid	A bid price is a price offered by a buyer when he/she buys a good. In the context of stock trading on a stock exchange, the bid price is the highest price a buyer of a stock is willing to pay for a share of that given stock.
Capital loss	Capital loss refers to the loss in value that the owner of an asset experiences when the price of the asset falls, including when the currency in which the asset is denominated depreciates. Contrasts with capital gain.
Capital gain	Capital gain refers to the gain in value that the owner of an asset experiences when the price of the asset rises, including when the currency in which the asset is denominated appreciates.
Creditworthiness	Creditworthiness indicates whether a borrower has in the past made loan payments when due.
Yield to maturity	Yield to maturity refers to the required rate of return on a bond issue. It is the discount rate used in present-valuing future interest payments and the principal payment at maturity. The term is used interchangeably with market rate of interest.
Expected rate of return	Expected rate of return refers to the increase in profit a firm anticipates it will obtain by purchasing capital ; expressed as a percentage of the total cost of the investment activity.
Call price	Call price refers to specified price that must be paid for bonds that are called; usually higher than the face amount of the bonds.
Bond market	The bond market refers to people and entities involved in buying and selling of bonds and the quantity and prices of those transactions over time.
Holding	The holding is a court's determination of a matter of law based on the issue presented in the particular case. In other words: under this law, with these facts, this result.
Future value	Future value measures what money is worth at a specified time in the future assuming a certain interest rate. This is used in time value of money calculations.
Buyer	A buyer refers to a role in the buying center with formal authority and responsibility to select the supplier and negotiate the terms of the contract.
Interest rate risk	Interest rate risk is the risk that the relative value of a security, especially a bond, will worsen due to an interest rate increase. This risk is commonly measured by the bond's duration.
Matching	Matching refers to an accounting concept that establishes when expenses are recognized. Expenses are matched with the revenues they helped to generate and are recognized when those

Chapter 11. Long-Term Debt Financing

Chapter 11. Long-Term Debt Financing

	revenues are recognized.
Dividend	Amount of corporate profits paid out for each share of stock is referred to as dividend.
Bond indenture	Bond contract that specifies the stated rate of interest and the face value of the bond as well as other contractual provisions is called the bond indenture. A company's bond indenture will cover all bonds issued by that company and also list all bond covenants.
Current yield	Current yield refers to the rate of return on a bond; the annual interest payment divided by the bond's price.
At par	At equality refers to at par. Two currencies are said to be 'at par' if they are trading one-for-one.
Coupon bond	A credit market instrument, the coupon bond pays the owner a fixed interest payment every year until the maturity date, when a specified final amount is repaid.
Federal Reserve	The Federal Reserve System was created via the Federal Reserve Act of December 23rd, 1913. All national banks were required to join the system and other banks could join. The Reserve Banks opened for business on November 16th, 1914. Federal Reserve Notes were created as part of the legislation, to provide an elastic supply of currency.
Financial management	The job of managing a firm's resources so it can meet its goals and objectives is called financial management.
Management	Management characterizes the process of leading and directing all or part of an organization, often a business, through the deployment and manipulation of resources. Early twentieth-century management writer Mary Parker Follett defined management as "the art of getting things done through people."
Bearer bond	A bearer bond is a legal certificate that usually represents a bond obligation of, or stock in, a corporation or some other intangible property.
Bearer	A person in possession of a negotiable instrument that is payable to him, his order, or to whoever is in possession of the instrument is referred to as bearer.
Registered bond	A registered bond refers to a bond for which the issuing company keeps a record of the name and address of the bondholder and pays interest and principal payments directly to the registered owner.
Agent	A person who makes economic decisions for another economic actor. A hired manager operates as an agent for a firm's owner.
Zero coupon bond	A zero coupon bond is a bond which do not pay periodic coupons, or so-called "interest payments." They are purchased at a discount from their value at maturity. The holder of a zero coupon bond is entitled to receive a single payment, usually of a specified sum of money at a specified time in the future.
Credit risk	The risk of loss due to a counterparty defaulting on a contract, or more generally the risk of loss due to some "credit event" is called credit risk.
Industry	A group of firms that produce identical or similar products is an industry. It is also used specifically to refer to an area of economic production focused on manufacturing which involves large amounts of capital investment before any profit can be realized, also called "heavy industry".
Option	A contract that gives the purchaser the option to buy or sell the underlying financial instrument at a specified price, called the exercise price or strike price, within a specific period of time.
Primary market	The market for the raising of new funds as opposed to the trading of securities already in

Go to **Cram101.com** for the Practice Tests for this Chapter.

Chapter 11. Long-Term Debt Financing

Chapter 11. Long-Term Debt Financing

	existence is called primary market.
Derivative	A derivative is a generic term for specific types of investments from which payoffs over time are derived from the performance of assets (such as commodities, shares or bonds), interest rates, exchange rates, or indices (such as a stock market index, consumer price index (CPI) or an index of weather conditions).
Tax reform	Tax reform is the process of changing the way taxes are collected or managed by the government. Some seek to reduce the level of taxation of all people by the government. Some seek to make the tax system more/less progressive in its effect. Some may be trying to make the tax system more understandable, or more accountable.
Tax Reform Act of 1986	Tax legislation that eliminated many of the abuses in the tax code and, at the same time, lowered the overall tax rates is a Tax Reform Act of 1986.
Estate	An estate is the totality of the legal rights, interests, entitlements and obligations attaching to property. In the context of wills and probate, it refers to the totality of the property which the deceased owned or in which some interest was held.
Swap	In finance a swap is a derivative, where two counterparties exchange one stream of cash flows against another stream. These streams are called the legs of the swap. The cash flows are calculated over a notional principal amount. Swaps are often used to hedge certain risks, for instance interest rate risk. Another use is speculation.
Trend	Trend refers to the long-term movement of an economic variable, such as its average rate of increase or decrease over enough years to encompass several business cycles.

Chapter 11. Long-Term Debt Financing

Chapter 12. Equity Financing

Common stock	Common stock refers to the basic, normal, voting stock issued by a corporation; called residual equity because it ranks after preferred stock for dividend and liquidation distributions.
Valuation	In finance, valuation is the process of estimating the market value of a financial asset or liability. They can be done on assets (for example, investments in marketable securities such as stocks, options, business enterprises, or intangible assets such as patents and trademarks) or on liabilities (e.g., Bonds issued by a company).
Stock	In financial terminology, stock is the capital raized by a corporation, through the issuance and sale of shares.
Market	A market is, as defined in economics, a social arrangement that allows buyers and sellers to discover information and carry out a voluntary exchange of goods or services.
Equity financing	Financing that consists of funds that are invested in exchange for ownership in the company is called equity financing.
Equity	Equity is the name given to the set of legal principles, in countries following the English common law tradition, which supplement strict rules of law where their application would operate harshly, so as to achieve what is sometimes referred to as "natural justice."
Firm	An organization that employs resources to produce a good or service for profit and owns and operates one or more plants is referred to as a firm.
Contribution	In business organization law, the cash or property contributed to a business by its owners is referred to as contribution.
Capital	Capital generally refers to financial wealth, especially that used to start or maintain a business. In classical economics, capital is one of four factors of production, the others being land and labor and entrepreneurship.
Grant	Grant refers to an intergovernmental transfer of funds . Since the New Deal, state and local governments have become increasingly dependent upon federal grants for an almost infinite variety of programs.
Fund	Independent accounting entity with a self-balancing set of accounts segregated for the purposes of carrying on specific activities is referred to as a fund.
Financial perspective	Financial perspective is one of the four standard perspectives used with the Balanced Scorecard. Financial perspective measures inform an organization whether strategy execution, which is detailed through measures in the other three perspectives, is leading to improved bottom line results.
Investment	Investment refers to spending for the production and accumulation of capital and additions to inventories. In a financial sense, buying an asset with the expectation of making a return.
Security	Security refers to a claim on the borrower future income that is sold by the borrower to the lender. A security is a type of transferable interest representing financial value.
Interest	In finance and economics, interest is the price paid by a borrower for the use of a lender's money. In other words, interest is the amount of paid to "rent" money for a period of time.
Stockholder	A stockholder is an individual or company (including a corporation) that legally owns one or more shares of stock in a joined stock company. The shareholders are the owners of a corporation. Companies listed at the stock market strive to enhance shareholder value.
Corporation	A legal entity chartered by a state or the Federal government that is distinct and separate from the individuals who own it is a corporation. This separation gives the corporation unique powers which other legal entities lack.

Go to Cram101.com for the Practice Tests for this Chapter.

Chapter 12. Equity Financing

Chapter 12. Equity Financing

Privilege	Generally, a legal right to engage in conduct that would otherwise result in legal liability is a privilege. Privileges are commonly classified as absolute or conditional. Occasionally, privilege is also used to denote a legal right to refrain from particular behavior.
Residual	Residual payments can refer to an ongoing stream of payments in respect of the completion of past achievements.
Gain	In finance, gain is a profit or an increase in value of an investment such as a stock or bond. Gain is calculated by fair market value or the proceeds from the sale of the investment minus the sum of the purchase price and all costs associated with it.
Net income	Net income is equal to the income that a firm has after subtracting costs and expenses from the total revenue. Expenses will typically include tax expense.
Expense	In accounting, an expense represents an event in which an asset is used up or a liability is incurred. In terms of the accounting equation, expenses reduce owners' equity.
Dividend	Amount of corporate profits paid out for each share of stock is referred to as dividend.
Asset	An item of property, such as land, capital, money, a share in ownership, or a claim on others for future payment, such as a bond or a bank deposit is an asset.
Cash dividend	A pro rata distribution of cash to stockholders of corporate stock is called a cash dividend.
Cash flow	In finance, cash flow refers to the amounts of cash being received and spent by a business during a defined period of time, sometimes tied to a specific project. Most of the time they are being used to determine gaps in the liquid position of a company.
Common stockholder	A person who owns common stock is referred to as common stockholder. They elect the members of the board of directors for the company, as well.
Board of directors	The group of individuals elected by the stockholders of a corporation to oversee its operations is a board of directors.
Chief executive officer	A chief executive officer is the highest-ranking corporate officer or executive officer of a corporation, or agency. In closely held corporations, it is general business culture that the office chief executive officer is also the chairman of the board.
Holding	The holding is a court's determination of a matter of law based on the issue presented in the particular case. In other words: under this law, with these facts, this result.
Shares	Shares refer to an equity security, representing a shareholder's ownership of a corporation. Shares are one of a finite number of equal portions in the capital of a company, entitling the owner to a proportion of distributed, non-reinvested profits known as dividends and to a portion of the value of the company in case of liquidation.
Proxy	Proxy refers to a person who is authorized to vote the shares of another person. Also, the written authorization empowering a person to vote the shares of another person.
Management	Management characterizes the process of leading and directing all or part of an organization, often a business, through the deployment and manipulation of resources. Early twentieth-century management writer Mary Parker Follett defined management as "the art of getting things done through people."
Takeover	A takeover in business refers to one company (the acquirer) purchasing another (the target). Such events resemble mergers, but without the formation of a new company.
Poison pill	Poison pill refers to a strategy that makes a firm unattractive as a potential takeover candidate. These are attempts by a potential acquirer to obtain a control block of shares in a target company, and thereby gain control of the board and, through it, the company's management.

Chapter 12. Equity Financing

Chapter 12. Equity Financing

Charter	Charter refers to an instrument or authority from the sovereign power bestowing the right or power to do business under the corporate form of organization. Also, the organic law of a city or town, and representing a portion of the statute law of the state.
Tactic	A short-term immediate decision that, in its totality, leads to the achievement of strategic goals is called a tactic.
Shareholder	A shareholder is an individual or company (including a corporation) that legally owns one or more shares of stock in a joined stock company.
Preemptive right	Preemptive right refers to a shareholder's option to purchase new issuances of shares in proportion to the shareholder's current ownership of the corporation.
Purchasing	Purchasing refers to the function in a firm that searches for quality material resources, finds the best suppliers, and negotiates the best price for goods and services.
Profit	Profit refers to the return to the resource entrepreneurial ability; total revenue minus total cost.
Retained earnings	Cumulative earnings of a company that are not distributed to the owners and are reinvested in the business are called retained earnings.
A share	In finance the term A share has two distinct meanings, both relating to securities. The first is a designation for a 'class' of common or preferred stock. A share of common or preferred stock typically has enhanced voting rights or other benefits compared to the other forms of shares that may have been created. The equity structure, or how many types of shares are offered, is determined by the corporate charter.
Rights offering	A rights offering is an offering of common stock to existing shareholders who hold subscription rights or pre-emptive rights that entitle them to buy newly issued shares at a discount from the price at which they will be offered to the public later
Issued shares	Issued shares refer to the number of shares that a corporation has sold to its shareholders. This may be equal to or less than the number of shares a company is authorized to issue.
Market price	Market price is an economic concept with commonplace familiarity; it is the price that a good or service is offered at, or will fetch, in the marketplace; it is of interest mainly in the study of microeconomics.
Holder	A person in possession of a document of title or an instrument payable or indorsed to him, his order, or to bearer is a holder.
Option	A contract that gives the purchaser the option to buy or sell the underlying financial instrument at a specified price, called the exercise price or strike price, within a specific period of time.
Private placement	Private placement refers to the sale of securities directly to a financial institution by a corporation. This eliminates the middleman and reduces the cost of issue to the corporation.
Institutional investors	Institutional investors refers to large organizations such as pension funds, mutual funds, insurance companies, and banks that invest their own funds or the funds of others.
Pension fund	Amounts of money put aside by corporations, nonprofit organizations, or unions to cover part of the financial needs of members when they retire is a pension fund.
Mutual fund	A mutual fund is a form of collective investment that pools money from many investors and invests the money in stocks, bonds, short-term money market instruments, and/or other securities. In a mutual fund, the fund manager trades the fund's underlying securities, realizing capital gains or loss, and collects the dividend or interest income.
Insurance	Insurance refers to a system by which individuals can reduce their exposure to risk of large

Go to Cram101.com for the Practice Tests for this Chapter.

Chapter 12. Equity Financing

Chapter 12. Equity Financing

	losses by spreading the risks among a large number of persons.
Pension	A pension is a steady income given to a person (usually after retirement). Pensions are typically payments made in the form of a guaranteed annuity to a retired or disabled employee.
Issuer	The company that borrows money from investors by issuing bonds is referred to as issuer. They are legally responsible for the obligations of the issue and for reporting financial conditions, material developments and any other operational activities as required by the regulations of their jurisdictions.
Stock purchase plan	A stock purchase plan is an organized plan for employees of a company to buy shares of its stock.
Stock option	A stock option is a specific type of option that uses the stock itself as an underlying instrument to determine the option's pay-off and therefore its value.
Incentive	An incentive is any factor (financial or non-financial) that provides a motive for a particular course of action, or counts as a reason for preferring one choice to the alternatives.
Incentive stock option	Incentive stock option refers to a type of stock option that receives favorable tax treatment. If various qualification requirements can be satisfied, there are no recognition tax consequences when the stock option is granted.
Discount	The difference between the face value of a bond and its selling price, when a bond is sold for less than its face value it's referred to as a discount.
Issued stock	The actual number of shares of stock currently classified as issued-comprises all the shares given in return for ownership in the corporation less any shares that have been retired is called issued stock.
Open market	In economics, the open market is the term used to refer to the environment in which bonds are bought and sold.
Allocate	Allocate refers to the assignment of income for various tax purposes. A multistate corporation's nonbusiness income usually is distributed to the state where the nonbusiness assets are located; it is not apportioned with the rest of the entity's income.
Pro rata	Proportionate is referred to as pro rata. A method of equally and proportionately allocating money, profits or liabilities by percentage.
Trustee	An independent party appointed to represent the bondholders is referred to as a trustee.
Consumption	In Keynesian economics consumption refers to personal consumption expenditure, i.e., the purchase of currently produced goods and services out of income, out of savings (net worth), or from borrowed funds. It refers to that part of disposable income that does not go to saving.
Investment banker	Investment banker refers to a financial organization that specializes in selling primary offerings of securities. Investment bankers can also perform other financial functions, such as advising clients, negotiating mergers and takeovers, and selling secondary offerings.
Debit	Debit refers to recording as negative in the balance of payments, any transaction that gives rise to a payment out of the country, such as an import, the purchase of an asset, or lending to foreigners. Opposite of credit.
Exchange	The trade of things of value between buyer and seller so that each is better off after the trade is called the exchange.
Stock exchange	A stock exchange is a corporation or mutual organization which provides facilities for stock

Chapter 12. Equity Financing

Chapter 12. Equity Financing

	brokers and traders, to trade company stocks and other securities.
Stock market	An organized marketplace in which common stocks are traded. In the United States, the largest stock market is the New York Stock Exchange, on which are traded the stocks of the largest U.S. companies.
Initial public offering	Firms in the process of becoming publicly traded companies will issue shares of stock using an initial public offering, which is merely the process of selling stock for the first time to interested investors.
Primary market	The market for the raising of new funds as opposed to the trading of securities already in existence is called primary market.
Secondary market	Secondary market refers to the market for securities that have already been issued. It is a market in which investors trade back and forth with each other.
Securities and exchange commission	Securities and exchange commission refers to U.S. government agency that determines the financial statements that public companies must provide to stockholders and the measurement rules that they must use in producing those statements.
Securities market	The securities market is the market for securities, where companies and the government can raise long-term funds.
Federal Reserve	The Federal Reserve System was created via the Federal Reserve Act of December 23rd, 1913. All national banks were required to join the system and other banks could join. The Reserve Banks opened for business on November 16th, 1914. Federal Reserve Notes were created as part of the legislation, to provide an elastic supply of currency.
Regulation	Regulation refers to restrictions state and federal laws place on business with regard to the conduct of its activities.
Prospectus	Prospectus refers to a report detailing a future stock offering containing a set of financial statements; required by the SEC from a company that wishes to make an initial public offering of its stock.
Registration statement	Document that an issuer of securities files with the SEC that contains required information about the issuer, the securities to be issued, and other relevant information so the security may be sold on a national stock exchange is a registration statement.
Red herring	Red herring prospectus is an initial prospectus to be submitted by a company which issues IPO. This prospectus has to be filed with SEC.It containing all the information about the company except for the offer price and the effective date, which aren't known at that time.
Buyer	A buyer refers to a role in the buying center with formal authority and responsibility to select the supplier and negotiate the terms of the contract.
Final prospectus	A final version of the prospectus that must be delivered by the issuer to the investor prior to or at the time of confirming a sale or sending a security to a purchaser is referred to as final prospectus.
Misrepresenttion	The assertion of a fact that is not in accord with the truth is misrepresentation. A contract can be rescinded on the ground of misrepresentation when the assertion relates to a material fact or is made fraudulently and the other party actually and justifiably relies on the assertion.
Damages	The sum of money recoverable by a plaintiff who has received a judgment in a civil case is called damages.
Underwriters	Investment banks that guarantee prices on securities to corporations and then sell the securities to the public are underwriters.

Go to Cram101.com for the Practice Tests for this Chapter.

Chapter 12. Equity Financing

Chapter 12. Equity Financing

Preparation	Preparation refers to usually the first stage in the creative process. It includes education and formal training.
Wash sale	A loss from the sale of stock or securities that is disallowed because the taxpayer, within 30 days before or after the sale, has acquired stock or securities substantially identical to those sold is a wash sale.
Margin requirement	Margin requirement refers to a rule that specifies the amount of cash or equity that must be deposited with a brokerage firm or bank, with the balance of funds eligible for borrowing. Margin is set by the Board of Governors of the Federal Reserve Board.
Credit	Credit refers to a recording as positive in the balance of payments, any transaction that gives rise to a payment into the country, such as an export, the sale of an asset, or borrowing from abroad.
Margin	A deposit by a buyer in stocks with a seller or a stockbroker, as security to cover fluctuations in the market in reference to stocks that the buyer has purchased but for which he has not paid is a margin. Commodities are also traded on margin.
Broker	In commerce, a broker is a party that mediates between a buyer and a seller. A broker who also acts as a seller or as a buyer becomes a principal party to the deal.
Blue sky laws	Blue sky laws are state (as opposed to federal) laws intended to protect investors against fraudulent securities practices. They typically require registration of offerings and licensing of participants.
Promoter	A person who incorporates a business, organizes its initial management, and raises its initial capital is a promoter.
Brokerage firm	A company that conducts various aspects of securities trading, analysis and advisory services is a brokerage firm.
Industry	A group of firms that produce identical or similar products is an industry. It is also used specifically to refer to an area of economic production focused on manufacturing which involves large amounts of capital investment before any profit can be realized, also called "heavy industry".
Investment banks	Investment banks, assist public and private corporations in raising funds in the capital markets (both equity and debt), as well as in providing strategic advisory services for mergers, acquisitions and other types of financial transactions. They also act as intermediaries in trading for clients. Investment banks differ from commercial banks, which take deposits and make commercial and retail loans.
Merrill Lynch	Merrill Lynch through its subsidiaries and affiliates, provides capital markets services, investment banking and advisory services, wealth management, asset management, insurance, banking and related products and services on a global basis. It is best known for its Global Private Client services and its strong sales force.
Best efforts	Best efforts refer to a distribution in which the investment banker agrees to work for a commission rather than actually underwriting the issue for resale. It is a procedure that is used by smaller investment bankers with relatively unknown companies. The investment banker is not directly taking the risk for distribution.
Bond	Bond refers to a debt instrument, issued by a borrower and promising a specified stream of payments to the purchaser, usually regular interest payments plus a final repayment of principal.
Fixed cost	The cost that a firm bears if it does not produce at all and that is independent of its output. The presence of a fixed cost tends to imply increasing returns to scale. Contrasts with variable cost.

Go to Cram101.com for the Practice Tests for this Chapter.

Chapter 12. Equity Financing

Chapter 12. Equity Financing

Yield to maturity	Yield to maturity refers to the required rate of return on a bond issue. It is the discount rate used in present-valuing future interest payments and the principal payment at maturity. The term is used interchangeably with market rate of interest.
Maturity	Maturity refers to the final payment date of a loan or other financial instrument, after which point no further interest or principal need be paid.
Yield	The interest rate that equates a future value or an annuity to a given present value is a yield.
Conflict of interest	A conflict that occurs when a corporate officer or director enters into a transaction with the corporation in which he or she has a personal interest is a conflict of interest.
Distribution	Distribution in economics, the manner in which total output and income is distributed among individuals or factors.
Underwriting	The process of selling securities and, at the same time, assuring the seller a specified price is underwriting. Underwriting is done by investment bankers and represents a form of risk taking.
Underwriting syndicate	Underwriting syndicate refers to a group of investment bankers that is formed to share the risk of a security offering and also to facilitate the distribution of the securities.
Dealer	People who link buyers with sellers by buying and selling securities at stated prices are referred to as a dealer.
Equity capital	Equity capital refers to money raized from within the firm or through the sale of ownership in the firm.
Charitable contributions	Charitable contributions refers to contributions that are tax deductible if made to qualified nonprofit charitable organizations. A cash basis taxpayer is entitled to a deduction solely in the year of payment.
Service	Service refers to a "non tangible product" that is not embodied in a physical good and that typically effects some change in another product, person, or institution. Contrasts with good.
Deductible	The dollar sum of costs that an insured individual must pay before the insurer begins to pay is called deductible.
Pledge	In law a pledge (also pawn) is a bailment of personal property as a security for some debt or engagement.
Stock valuation	There are several methods used for stock valuation. They try to give an estimate of their fair value, by using fundamental economic criteria. This theoretical valuation has to be perfected with market criteria, as the final purpose is to determine potential market prices.
Cash flow forecast	Forecast that predicts the cash inflows and outflows in future periods is a cash flow forecast. It is a company's projected cash receipts and disbursements over a set time horizon.
Present value	The value today of a stream of payments and/or receipts over time in the future and/or the past, converted to the present using an interest rate. If X_t is the amount in period t and r the interest rate, then present value at time t=0 is $V = ?T /t$.
Dividend valuation model	A model for determining the value of a share of stock by taking the present value of an expected stream of future dividends is referred to as dividend valuation model.
Dividend yield	Dividends per share divided by market price per share are called a dividend yield. Dividend yield indicates the percentage return that a stockholder will receive on dividends alone.
Capital gain	Capital gain refers to the gain in value that the owner of an asset experiences when the price of the asset rises, including when the currency in which the asset is denominated

Chapter 12. Equity Financing

Chapter 12. Equity Financing

	appreciates.
Liquidated	Damages made certain by the prior agreement of the parties are called liquidated.
Controlling interest	A firm has a controlling interest in another business entity when it owns more than 50 percent of that entity's voting stock.
Outstanding stock	Outstanding stock refers to capital stock that has been issued and is being held by stockholders.
Controlling	A management function that involves determining whether or not an organization is progressing toward its goals and objectives, and taking corrective action if it is not is called controlling.
Bid	A bid price is a price offered by a buyer when he/she buys a good. In the context of stock trading on a stock exchange, the bid price is the highest price a buyer of a stock is willing to pay for a share of that given stock.
Rate of return	A rate of return is a comparison of the money earned (or lost) on an investment to the amount of money invested.
Required rate of return	Required rate of return refers to the rate of return that investors demand from an investment to compensate them for the amount of risk involved.
Earnings per share	Earnings per share refers to annual profit of the corporation divided by the number of shares outstanding.
Inflation rate	The percentage increase in the price level per year is an inflation rate. Alternatively, the inflation rate is the rate of decrease in the purchasing power of money.
Inflation	An increase in the overall price level of an economy, usually as measured by the CPI or by the implicit price deflator is called inflation.
Economy	The income, expenditures, and resources that affect the cost of running a business and household are called an economy.
Productive assets	Productive assets refers to assets used to operate the business; frequently called long-term assets. They are property such as land, livestock, and trees that produce income.
Expected rate of return	Expected rate of return refers to the increase in profit a firm anticipates it will obtain by purchasing capital; expressed as a percentage of the total cost of the investment activity.
Scope	Scope of a project is the sum total of all projects products and their requirements or features.
Interest rate	The rate of return on bonds, loans, or deposits. When one speaks of 'the' interest rate, it is usually in a model where there is only one.
Efficient market	Efficient market refers to a market in which, at a minimum, current price changes are independent of past price changes, or, more strongly, price reflects all available information.
Inside information	Confidential information of a company, its products, or securities not generally available to the public gained from a source inside the company is called inside information.
Abnormal returns	Abnormal returns is a term used by stock market traders to describe the difference between a single stock or portfolio's performance in regard to the average market performance (usually a broad index s.a. the S&P 500 and EURO STOXX 50 or a national index like the Nikkei) over a set period of time.
Treasury security	A treasury security is a government bond issued by the United States Department of the Treasury through the Bureau of the Public Debt. They are the debt financing instruments of

Go to Cram101.com for the Practice Tests for this Chapter.

Chapter 12. Equity Financing

Chapter 12. Equity Financing

	the U.S. Federal government, and are often referred to simply as Treasuries.
Analyst	Analyst refers to a person or tool with a primary function of information analysis, generally with a more limited, practical and short term set of goals than a researcher.
Abnormal profit	Abnormal profit is an economic term of profit exceeding the normal profit. Normal profit equals the opportunity cost of labor and capital, while supernormal profit is the amount exceeds the normal return from these input factors in production.
Research and development	The use of resources for the deliberate discovery of new information and ways of doing things, together with the application of that information in inventing new products or processes is referred to as research and development.
Long run	In economic models, the long run time frame assumes no fixed factors of production. Firms can enter or leave the marketplace, and the cost (and availability) of land, labor, raw materials, and capital goods can be assumed to vary.
Future interest	Future interest refers to an interest that will come into being at some future time. It is distinguished from a present interest, which already exists. Assume that Dan transfers securities to a newly created trust.
Expected return	Expected return refers to the return on an asset expected over the next period.
Cost of equity	In finance, the cost of equity is the minimum rate of return a firm must offer shareholders to compensate for waiting for their returns, and for bearing some risk.
Closely held corporation	Closely held corporation refers to a corporation where stock ownership is not widely dispersed. Rather, a few shareholders are in control of corporate policy and are in a position to benefit personally from that policy.
Enterprise	Enterprise refers to another name for a business organization. Other similar terms are business firm, sometimes simply business, sometimes simply firm, as well as company, and entity.
Market risk premium	Market risk premium refers to a premium over and above the risk-free rate. It is represented by the difference between the market return and the risk-free rate, and it may be multiplied by the beta coefficient to determine the additional risk-adjusted return on a security.
Risk premium	In finance, the risk premium can be the expected rate of return above the risk-free interest rate.
Market risk	Market risk is the risk that the value of an investment will decrease due to moves in market factors.
Premium	Premium refers to the fee charged by an insurance company for an insurance policy. The rate of losses must be relatively predictable: In order to set the premium (prices) insurers must be able to estimate them accurately.
Rate of return on investment	The rate of return on investment refers to the benefits to an investor (the profit) relative to the cost of the initial investment.
Return on investment	Return on investment refers to the return a businessperson gets on the money he and other owners invest in the firm; for example, a business that earned $100 on a $1,000 investment would have a ROI of 10 percent: 100 divided by 1000.
Ambulatory care	Ambulatory care is any medical care delivered on an outpatient basis. Many medical conditions do not require hospital admission and can be managed without admission to a hospital. Many medical investigations can be performed on an ambulatory basis, including blood tests, X-rays, endoscopy and even biopsy procedures of superficial organs.
Preferred stock	Stock that has specified rights over common stock is a preferred stock.

Go to **Cram101.com** for the Practice Tests for this Chapter.

Chapter 12. Equity Financing

Chapter 12. Equity Financing

Administrative cost	An administrative cost is all executive, organizational, and clerical costs associated with the general management of an organization rather than with manufacturing, marketing, or selling
Wall Street Journal	Dow Jones & Company was founded in 1882 by reporters Charles Dow, Edward Jones and Charles Bergstresser. Jones converted the small Customers' Afternoon Letter into The Wall Street Journal, first published in 1889, and began delivery of the Dow Jones News Service via telegraph. The Journal featured the Jones 'Average', the first of several indexes of stock and bond prices on the New York Stock Exchange.
Advertisement	Advertisement is the promotion of goods, services, companies and ideas, usually by an identified sponsor. Marketers see advertising as part of an overall promotional strategy.
Journal	Book of original entry, in which transactions are recorded in a general ledger system, is referred to as a journal.
Reorganization	Reorganization occurs, among other instances, when one corporation acquires another in a merger or acquisition, a single corporation divides into two or more entities, or a corporation makes a substantial change in its capital structure.
Conversion	Conversion refers to any distinct act of dominion wrongfully exerted over another's personal property in denial of or inconsistent with his rights therein. That tort committed by a person who deals with chattels not belonging to him in a manner that is inconsistent with the ownership of the lawful owner.

Chapter 12. Equity Financing

Chapter 13. Capital Structure and the Cost of Capital

Equity financing	Financing that consists of funds that are invested in exchange for ownership in the company is called equity financing.
Equity	Equity is the name given to the set of legal principles, in countries following the English common law tradition, which supplement strict rules of law where their application would operate harshly, so as to achieve what is sometimes referred to as "natural justice."
Cost of capital	Cost of capital refers to the percentage cost of funds used for acquiring resources for an organization, typically a weighted average of the firms cost of equity and cost of debt.
Capital	Capital generally refers to financial wealth, especially that used to start or maintain a business. In classical economics, capital is one of four factors of production, the others being land and labor and entrepreneurship.
Investment	Investment refers to spending for the production and accumulation of capital and additions to inventories. In a financial sense, buying an asset with the expectation of making a return.
Capital structure	Capital Structure refers to the way a corporation finances itself through some combination of equity sales, equity options, bonds, and loans. Optimal capital structure refers to the particular combination that minimizes the cost of capital while maximizing the stock price.
Balance sheet	A statement of the assets, liabilities, and net worth of a firm or individual at some given time often at the end of its "fiscal year," is referred to as a balance sheet.
Liability	A liability is a present obligation of the enterprise arizing from past events, the settlement of which is expected to result in an outflow from the enterprise of resources embodying economic benefits.
Balance	In banking and accountancy, the outstanding balance is the amount of money owned, (or due), that remains in a deposit account (or a loan account) at a given date, after all past remittances, payments and withdrawal have been accounted for. It can be positive (then, in the balance sheet of a firm, it is an asset) or negative (a liability).
Financial statement	Financial statement refers to a summary of all the transactions that have occurred over a particular period.
Debt financing	Obtaining financing by borrowing money is debt financing.
Accounting	A system that collects and processes financial information about an organization and reports that information to decision makers is referred to as accounting.
Common stock	Common stock refers to the basic, normal, voting stock issued by a corporation; called residual equity because it ranks after preferred stock for dividend and liquidation distributions.
Stock	In financial terminology, stock is the capital raized by a corporation, through the issuance and sale of shares.
Current asset	A current asset is an asset on the balance sheet which is expected to be sold or otherwise used up in the near future, usually within one year.
Fixed asset	Fixed asset, also known as property, plant, and equipment (PP&E), is a term used in accountancy for assets and property which cannot easily be converted into cash. This can be compared with current assets such as cash or bank accounts, which are described as liquid assets. In most cases, only tangible assets are referred to as fixed.
Operation	A standardized method or technique that is performed repetitively, often on different materials resulting in different finished goods is called an operation.
Asset	An item of property, such as land, capital, money, a share in ownership, or a claim on others for future payment, such as a bond or a bank deposit is an asset.

Go to **Cram101.com** for the Practice Tests for this Chapter.

Chapter 13. Capital Structure and the Cost of Capital

Chapter 13. Capital Structure and the Cost of Capital

Interest rate	The rate of return on bonds, loans, or deposits. When one speaks of 'the' interest rate, it is usually in a model where there is only one.
Creditor	A person to whom a debt or legal obligation is owed, and who has the right to enforce payment of that debt or obligation is referred to as creditor.
Interest	In finance and economics, interest is the price paid by a borrower for the use of a lender's money. In other words, interest is the amount of paid to "rent" money for a period of time.
Operating income	Total revenues from operation minus cost of goods sold and operating costs are called operating income.
Revenue	Revenue is a U.S. business term for the amount of money that a company receives from its activities, mostly from sales of products and/or services to customers.
Firm	An organization that employs resources to produce a good or service for profit and owns and operates one or more plants is referred to as a firm.
Income statement	Income statement refers to a financial statement that presents the revenues and expenses and resulting net income or net loss of a company for a specific period of time.
Equity investment	Equity investment generally refers to the buying and holding of shares of stock on a stock market by individuals and funds in anticipation of income from dividends and capital gain as the value of the stock rises.
Net income	Net income is equal to the income that a firm has after subtracting costs and expenses from the total revenue. Expenses will typically include tax expense.
Return on equity	Net profit after taxes per dollar of equity capital is referred to as return on equity.
Rate of return	A rate of return is a comparison of the money earned (or lost) on an investment to the amount of money invested.
Book value	The book value of an asset or group of assets is sometimes the price at which they were originally acquired, in many cases equal to purchase price.
Capital requirement	The capital requirement is a bank regulation, which sets a framework on how banks and depository institutions must handle their capital. The categorization of assets and capital is highly standardized so that it can be risk weighted.
Bottom line	The bottom line is net income on the last line of a income statement.
Expected rate of return	Expected rate of return refers to the increase in profit a firm anticipates it will obtain by purchasing capital ; expressed as a percentage of the total cost of the investment activity.
Financial leverage	A measure of the amount of debt used in the capital structure of the firm is the financial leverage.
Leverage	Leverage is using given resources in such a way that the potential positive or negative outcome is magnified. In finance, this generally refers to borrowing.
Distribution	Distribution in economics, the manner in which total output and income is distributed among individuals or factors.
Standard deviation	A measure of the spread or dispersion of a series of numbers around the expected value is the standard deviation. The standard deviation tells us how well the expected value represents a series of values.
Capital structure theory	A theory that addresses the relative importance of debt and equity in the overall financing of the firm is called capital structure theory.
Debt service	The payments made by a borrower on their debt, usually including both interest payments and

Go to **Cram101.com** for the Practice Tests for this Chapter.

Chapter 13. Capital Structure and the Cost of Capital

Chapter 13. Capital Structure and the Cost of Capital

	partial repayment of principal, are called debt service.
Service	Service refers to a "non tangible product" that is not embodied in a physical good and that typically effects some change in another product, person, or institution. Contrasts with good.
Default	In finance, default occurs when a debtor has not met its legal obligations according to the debt contract, e.g. it has not made a scheduled payment, or violated a covenant (condition) of the debt contract.
Lender	Suppliers and financial institutions that lend money to companies is referred to as a lender.
Cost of equity	In finance, the cost of equity is the minimum rate of return a firm must offer shareholders to compensate for waiting for their returns, and for bearing some risk.
Cost of debt	The cost of debt is the cost of borrowing money (usually denoted by Kd). It is derived by dividing debt's interest payments on the total market value of the debts.
Weighted average	The weighted average unit cost of the goods available for sale for both cost of goods sold and ending inventory.
Average cost	Average cost is equal to total cost divided by the number of goods produced (Quantity-Q). It is also equal to the sum of average variable costs (total variable costs divided by Q) plus average fixed costs (total fixed costs divided by Q).
Labor	People's physical and mental talents and efforts that are used to help produce goods and services are called labor.
Acquisition	A company's purchase of the property and obligations of another company is an acquisition.
Financial risk	The risk related to the inability of the firm to meet its debt obligations as they come due is called financial risk.
Business risk	The risk related to the inability of the firm to hold its competitive position and maintain stability and growth in earnings is business risk.
Inherent Risk	Inherent risk is the auditor's assessment that there are material misstatements in the financial statements before considering the effectiveness of internal controls. If the auditor concludes that there is a high likelihood of misstamtement, ignoring internal controls, the auditor would conclude that the inherent risk is high.
Return on Assets	The Return on Assets percentage shows how profitable a company's assets are in generating revenue.
Context	The effect of the background under which a message often takes on more and richer meaning is a context. Context is especially important in cross-cultural interactions because some cultures are said to be high context or low context.
Bond ratings	Bond ratings refers to rating of bonds according to risk by Standard & Poor's and Moody's Investor Service. A bond that is rated A by Moody's has the lowest risk, while a bond with a C rating has the highest risk. Coupon rates are greatly influenced by a corporation's bond rating.
Industry	A group of firms that produce identical or similar products is an industry. It is also used specifically to refer to an area of economic production focused on manufacturing which involves large amounts of capital investment before any profit can be realized, also called "heavy industry".
Bond	Bond refers to a debt instrument, issued by a borrower and promising a specified stream of payments to the purchaser, usually regular interest payments plus a final repayment of principal.

Chapter 13. Capital Structure and the Cost of Capital

Chapter 13. Capital Structure and the Cost of Capital

Management	Management characterizes the process of leading and directing all or part of an organization, often a business, through the deployment and manipulation of resources. Early twentieth-century management writer Mary Parker Follett defined management as "the art of getting things done through people."
Security	Security refers to a claim on the borrower future income that is sold by the borrower to the lender. A security is a type of transferable interest representing financial value.
Collateral	Property that is pledged to the lender to guarantee payment in the event that the borrower is unable to make debt payments is called collateral.
Retained earnings	Cumulative earnings of a company that are not distributed to the owners and are reinvested in the business are called retained earnings.
Fund	Independent accounting entity with a self-balancing set of accounts segregated for the purposes of carrying on specific activities is referred to as a fund.
Equity capital	Equity capital refers to money raized from within the firm or through the sale of ownership in the firm.
Contribution	In business organization law, the cash or property contributed to a business by its owners is referred to as contribution.
Proprietary	Proprietary indicates that a party, or proprietor, exercises private ownership, control or use over an item of property, usually to the exclusion of other parties. Where a party, holds or claims proprietary interests in relation to certain types of property (eg. a creative literary work, or software), that property may also be the subject of intellectual property law (eg. copyright or patents).
Market	A market is, as defined in economics, a social arrangement that allows buyers and sellers to discover information and carry out a voluntary exchange of goods or services.
Grant	Grant refers to an intergovernmental transfer of funds . Since the New Deal, state and local governments have become increasingly dependent upon federal grants for an almost infinite variety of programs.
Competitive advantage	A business is said to have a competitive advantage when its unique strengths, often based on cost, quality, time, and innovation, offer consumers a greater percieved value and there by differtiating it from its competitors.
Matching	Matching refers to an accounting concept that establishes when expenses are recognized. Expenses are matched with the revenues they helped to generate and are recognized when those revenues are recognized.
Cost structure	The relative proportion of an organization's fixed, variable, and mixed costs is referred to as cost structure.
Competitor	Other organizations in the same industry or type of business that provide a good or service to the same set of customers is referred to as a competitor.
Opportunity cost	The cost of something in terms of opportunity foregone. The opportunity cost to a country of producing a unit more of a good, such as for export or to replace an import, is the quantity of some other good that could have been produced instead.
Capital asset	In accounting, a capital asset is an asset that is recorded as property that creates more property, e.g. a factory that creates shoes, or a forest that yields a quantity of wood.
Marginal cost	Marginal cost refers to the increase in cost that accompanies a unit increase in output; the partial derivative of the cost function with respect to output.
Historical cost	In accounting terminology, historical cost describes the original cost of an asset at the

Chapter 13. Capital Structure and the Cost of Capital

Chapter 13. Capital Structure and the Cost of Capital

	time of purchase or payment as opposed to its market value
Debt capital	Debt capital refers to funds raized through various forms of borrowing to finance a company that must be repaid.
Investment banker	Investment banker refers to a financial organization that specializes in selling primary offerings of securities. Investment bankers can also perform other financial functions, such as advising clients, negotiating mergers and takeovers, and selling secondary offerings.
Interest payment	The payment to holders of bonds payable, calculated by multiplying the stated rate on the face of the bond by the par, or face, value of the bond. If bonds are issued at a discount or premium, the interest payment does not equal the interest expense.
Municipal bond	In the United States, a municipal bond is a bond issued by a state, city or other local government, or their agencies. Potential issuers of these include cities, counties, redevelopment agencies, school districts, publicly owned airports and seaports, and any other governmental entity (or group of governments) below the state level. They are guaranteed by a local government, a subdivision thereof, or a group of local governments, and are assessed for risk and rated accordingly.
Par value	The central value of a pegged exchange rate, around which the actual rate is permitted to fluctuate within set bounds is a par value.
Analyst	Analyst refers to a person or tool with a primary function of information analysis, generally with a more limited, practical and short term set of goals than a researcher.
Flotation cost	Flotation cost refers to the distribution cost of selling securities to the public. The cost includes the underwriter's spread and any associated fees.
Expense	In accounting, an expense represents an event in which an asset is used up or a liability is incurred. In terms of the accounting equation, expenses reduce owners' equity.
Yield to maturity	Yield to maturity refers to the required rate of return on a bond issue. It is the discount rate used in present-valuing future interest payments and the principal payment at maturity. The term is used interchangeably with market rate of interest.
Current yield	Current yield refers to the rate of return on a bond; the annual interest payment divided by the bond's price.
Maturity	Maturity refers to the final payment date of a loan or other financial instrument, after which point no further interest or principal need be paid.
Yield	The interest rate that equates a future value or an annuity to a given present value is a yield.
Yield curve	In finance, the yield curve is the relation between the interest rate (or cost of borrowing) and the maturity of the debt for a given borrower in a given currency.
Commercial bank	A firm that engages in the business of banking is a commercial bank.
Prime rate	The rate that a bank charges its most creditworthy customers is referred to as the prime rate.
Premium	Premium refers to the fee charged by an insurance company for an insurance policy. The rate of losses must be relatively predictable: In order to set the premium (prices) insurers must be able to estimate them accurately.
Shareholder	A shareholder is an individual or company (including a corporation) that legally owns one or more shares of stock in a joined stock company.
Dividend	Amount of corporate profits paid out for each share of stock is referred to as dividend.

Chapter 13. Capital Structure and the Cost of Capital

Chapter 13. Capital Structure and the Cost of Capital

Cost principle	A principle that holds that it is unethical to charge a higher price for a commodity than the cost of purchasing, producing or acquiring, and bringing it to market is the cost principle.
Common stockholder	A person who owns common stock is referred to as common stockholder. They elect the members of the board of directors for the company, as well.
Stockholder	A stockholder is an individual or company (including a corporation) that legally owns one or more shares of stock in a joined stock company. The shareholders are the owners of a corporation. Companies listed at the stock market strive to enhance shareholder value.
Bondholder	The individual or entity that purchases a bond, thus loaning money to the company that issued the bond is the bondholder.
Supply	Supply is the aggregate amount of any material good that can be called into being at a certain price point; it comprises one half of the equation of supply and demand. In classical economic theory, a curve representing supply is one of the factors that produce price.
Wage	The payment for the service of a unit of labor, per unit time. In trade theory, it is the only payment to labor, usually unskilled labor. In empirical work, wage data may exclude other compenzation, which must be added to get the total cost of employment.
Residual	Residual payments can refer to an ongoing stream of payments in respect of the completion of past achievements.
Commodity	Could refer to any good, but in trade a commodity is usually a raw material or primary product that enters into international trade, such as metals or basic agricultural products.
Futures	Futures refer to contracts for the sale and future delivery of stocks or commodities, wherein either party may waive delivery, and receive or pay, as the case may be, the difference in market price at the time set for delivery.
Estate	An estate is the totality of the legal rights, interests, entitlements and obligations attaching to property. In the context of wills and probate, it refers to the totality of the property which the deceased owned or in which some interest was held.
Required rate of return	Required rate of return refers to the rate of return that investors demand from an investment to compensate them for the amount of risk involved.
Shares	Shares refer to an equity security, representing a shareholder's ownership of a corporation. Shares are one of a finite number of equal portions in the capital of a company, entitling the owner to a proportion of distributed, non-reinvested profits known as dividends and to a portion of the value of the company in case of liquidation.
Capital asset pricing model	The capital asset pricing model is used in finance to determine a theoretically appropriate required rate of return (and thus the price if expected cash flows can be estimated) of an asset, if that asset is to be added to an already well-diversified portfolio, given that asset's non-diversifiable risk.
Discounted cash flow	In finance, the discounted cash flow approach describes a method to value a project or an entire company. The DCF methods determine the present value of future cash flows by discounting them using the appropriate cost of capital.
Risk premium	In finance, the risk premium can be the expected rate of return above the risk-free interest rate.
Cash flow	In finance, cash flow refers to the amounts of cash being received and spent by a business during a defined period of time, sometimes tied to a specific project. Most of the time they are being used to determine gaps in the liquid position of a company.
Treasury security	A treasury security is a government bond issued by the United States Department of the Treasury through the Bureau of the Public Debt. They are the debt financing instruments of

Go to **Cram101.com** for the Practice Tests for this Chapter.

Chapter 13. Capital Structure and the Cost of Capital

Chapter 13. Capital Structure and the Cost of Capital

	the U.S. Federal government, and are often referred to simply as Treasuries.
Default risk	The chance that the issuer of a debt instrument will be unable to make interest payments or pay off the face value when the instrument matures is called default risk.
Portfolio	In finance, a portfolio is a collection of investments held by an institution or a private individual. Holding but not always a portfolio is part of an investment and risk-limiting strategy called diversification. By owning several assets, certain types of risk (in particular specific risk) can be reduced.
Preference	The act of a debtor in paying or securing one or more of his creditors in a manner more favorable to them than to other creditors or to the exclusion of such other creditors is a preference. In the absence of statute, a preference is perfectly good, but to be legal it must be bona fide, and not a mere subterfuge of the debtor to secure a future benefit to himself or to prevent the application of his property to his debts.
Federal Reserve	The Federal Reserve System was created via the Federal Reserve Act of December 23rd, 1913. All national banks were required to join the system and other banks could join. The Reserve Banks opened for business on November 16th, 1914. Federal Reserve Notes were created as part of the legislation, to provide an elastic supply of currency.
Argument	The discussion by counsel for the respective parties of their contentions on the law and the facts of the case being tried in order to aid the jury in arriving at a correct and just conclusion is called argument.
Wall Street Journal	Dow Jones & Company was founded in 1882 by reporters Charles Dow, Edward Jones and Charles Bergstresser. Jones converted the small Customers' Afternoon Letter into The Wall Street Journal, first published in 1889, and began delivery of the Dow Jones News Service via telegraph. The Journal featured the Jones 'Average', the first of several indexes of stock and bond prices on the New York Stock Exchange.
Journal	Book of original entry, in which transactions are recorded in a general ledger system, is referred to as a journal.
Proxy	Proxy refers to a person who is authorized to vote the shares of another person. Also, the written authorization empowering a person to vote the shares of another person.
Market risk premium	Market risk premium refers to a premium over and above the risk-free rate. It is represented by the difference between the market return and the risk-free rate, and it may be multiplied by the beta coefficient to determine the additional risk-adjusted return on a security.
Expected return	Expected return refers to the return on an asset expected over the next period.
Market risk	Market risk is the risk that the value of an investment will decrease due to moves in market factors.
Derivative	A derivative is a generic term for specific types of investments from which payoffs over time are derived from the performance of assets (such as commodities, shares or bonds), interest rates, exchange rates, or indices (such as a stock market index, consumer price index (CPI) or an index of weather conditions).
Beta coefficient	The Beta coefficient (sensitivity of the asset returns to market returns, relative volatility), is a key parameter in the Capital asset pricing model. It can also be defined as the risk of the stock to a diversified portfolio.
Basis point	One one-hundredth of a percentage point is a basis point. Each one percent in interest is equal to 100 basis points.
Points	Loan origination fees that may be deductible as interest by a buyer of property. A seller of property who pays points reduces the selling price by the amount of the points paid for the

Go to Cram101.com for the Practice Tests for this Chapter.

Chapter 13. Capital Structure and the Cost of Capital

Chapter 13. Capital Structure and the Cost of Capital

	buyer.
Financial plan	The financial plan section of a business plan consists of three financial statements (the income statement, the cash flow projection, and the balance sheet) and a brief analysis of these three statements.
Present value	The value today of a stream of payments and/or receipts over time in the future and/or the past, converted to the present using an interest rate. If X_t is the amount in period t and r the interest rate, then present value at time t=0 is $V = ?T /t$.
Warrant	A warrant is a security that entitles the holder to buy or sell a certain additional quantity of an underlying security at an agreed-upon price, at the holder's discretion.
Marketable securities	Marketable securities refer to securities that are readily traded in the secondary securities market.
Debt ratio	Debt ratio refers to the calculation of the total liabilities divided by the total liabilities plus capital. This results in the measurment of the debt level of the business (leverage).
Depreciation	Depreciation is an accounting and finance term for the method of attributing the cost of an asset across the useful life of the asset. Depreciation is a reduction in the value of a currency in floating exchange rate.
Creditworthiness	Creditworthiness indicates whether a borrower has in the past made loan payments when due.
Marginal tax rate	The percentage of an additional dollar of earnings that goes to taxes is referred to as the marginal tax rate.
Closing	The finalization of a real estate sales transaction that passes title to the property from the seller to the buyer is referred to as a closing. Closing is a sales term which refers to the process of making a sale. It refers to reaching the final step, which may be an exchange of money or acquiring a signature.
Financial perspective	Financial perspective is one of the four standard perspectives used with the Balanced Scorecard. Financial perspective measures inform an organization whether strategy execution, which is detailed through measures in the other three perspectives, is leading to improved bottom line results.
Liquidated	Damages made certain by the prior agreement of the parties are called liquidated.
Consideration	Consideration in contract law, a basic requirement for an enforceable agreement under traditional contract principles, defined in this text as legal value, bargained for and given in exchange for an act or promise. In corporation law, cash or property contributed to a corporation in exchange for shares, or a promise to contribute such cash or property.
Subsidiary	A company that is controlled by another company or corporation is a subsidiary.
Hurdle rate	The minimum acceptable rate of return in a capital budgeting decision is the hurdle rate. The hurdle rate should reflect the riskiness of the investment, typically measured by volatility of cash flows, and must take into account the financing mix.
Financial analysis	Financial analysis is the analysis of the accounts and the economic prospects of a firm.
Corporation	A legal entity chartered by a state or the Federal government that is distinct and separate from the individuals who own it is a corporation. This separation gives the corporation unique powers which other legal entities lack.
Preferred stock	Stock that has specified rights over common stock is a preferred stock.
Inflation	An increase in the overall price level of an economy, usually as measured by the CPI or by

Chapter 13. Capital Structure and the Cost of Capital

Chapter 13. Capital Structure and the Cost of Capital

	the implicit price deflator is called inflation.
Volatility	Volatility refers to the extent to which an economic variable, such as a price or an exchange rate, moves up and down over time.
Variable	A variable is something measured by a number; it is used to analyze what happens to other things when the size of that number changes.
Dividend payout ratio	A measure of the percentage of earnings paid out in dividends; found by dividing cash dividends by the net income available to each class of stock is the dividend payout ratio.
Payout ratio	A measure of the percentage of earnings distributed in the form of cash dividends to common stockholders is referred to as the payout ratio. More specifically, the firm's cash dividend divided by the firm's earnings in the same reporting period.
Weighted average cost of capital	Weighted average cost of capital refers to the computed cost of capital determined by multiplying the cost of each item in the optimal capital structure by its weighted representation in the overall capital structure and summing up the results.
Financial management	The job of managing a firm's resources so it can meet its goals and objectives is called financial management.
Administration	Administration refers to the management and direction of the affairs of governments and institutions; a collective term for all policymaking officials of a government; the execution and implementation of public policy.
Market value	Market value refers to the price of an asset agreed on between a willing buyer and a willing seller; the price an asset could demand if it is sold on the open market.
Economics	The social science dealing with the use of scarce resources to obtain the maximum satisfaction of society's virtually unlimited economic wants is an economics.
Option	A contract that gives the purchaser the option to buy or sell the underlying financial instrument at a specified price, called the exercise price or strike price, within a specific period of time.
Nonprofit organization	An organization whose goals do not include making a personal profit for its owners is a nonprofit organization.
Policy	Similar to a script in that a policy can be a less than completely rational decision-making method. Involves the use of a pre-existing set of decision steps for any problem that presents itself.
Capital expenditure	A substantial expenditure that is used by a company to acquire or upgrade physical assets such as equipment, property, industrial buildings, including those which improve the quality and life of an asset is referred to as a capital expenditure.
Discount rate	Discount rate refers to the rate, per year, at which future values are diminished to make them comparable to values in the present. Can be either subjective or objective.
Discount	The difference between the face value of a bond and its selling price, when a bond is sold for less than its face value it's referred to as a discount.

Chapter 13. Capital Structure and the Cost of Capital

Chapter 14. The Basics of Capital Budgeting

Financial analysis	Financial analysis is the analysis of the accounts and the economic prospects of a firm.
Capital budgeting	Capital budgeting is the planning process used to determine a firm's long term investments such as new machinery, replacement machinery, new plants, new products, and research and development projects.
Service	Service refers to a "non tangible product" that is not embodied in a physical good and that typically effects some change in another product, person, or institution. Contrasts with good.
Capital	Capital generally refers to financial wealth, especially that used to start or maintain a business. In classical economics, capital is one of four factors of production, the others being land and labor and entrepreneurship.
Cash flow	In finance, cash flow refers to the amounts of cash being received and spent by a business during a defined period of time, sometimes tied to a specific project. Most of the time they are being used to determine gaps in the liquid position of a company.
Profitability analysis	A means of measuring the profitability of the firm's products, customer groups, sales territories, channels of distribution, and order sizes is called profitability analysis.
Capital structure	Capital Structure refers to the way a corporation finances itself through some combination of equity sales, equity options, bonds, and loans. Optimal capital structure refers to the particular combination that minimizes the cost of capital while maximizing the stock price.
Cost of capital	Cost of capital refers to the percentage cost of funds used for acquiring resources for an organization, typically a weighted average of the firms cost of equity and cost of debt.
Firm	An organization that employs resources to produce a good or service for profit and owns and operates one or more plants is referred to as a firm.
Incorporation	Incorporation is the forming of a new corporation. The corporation may be a business, a non-profit organization or even a government of a new city or town.
Fixed asset	Fixed asset, also known as property, plant, and equipment (PP&E), is a term used in accountancy for assets and property which cannot easily be converted into cash. This can be compared with current assets such as cash or bank accounts, which are described as liquid assets. In most cases, only tangible assets are referred to as fixed.
Asset	An item of property, such as land, capital, money, a share in ownership, or a claim on others for future payment, such as a bond or a bank deposit is an asset.
Competitor	Other organizations in the same industry or type of business that provide a good or service to the same set of customers is referred to as a competitor.
Technology	The body of knowledge and techniques that can be used to combine economic resources to produce goods and services is called technology.
Capital asset	In accounting, a capital asset is an asset that is recorded as property that creates more property, e.g. a factory that creates shoes, or a forest that yields a quantity of wood.
Acquisition	A company's purchase of the property and obligations of another company is an acquisition.
Procurement	Procurement is the acquisition of goods or services at the best possible total cost of ownership, in the right quantity, at the right time, in the right place for the direct benefit or use of the governments, corporations, or individuals generally via, but not limited to a contract.
Fund	Independent accounting entity with a self-balancing set of accounts segregated for the purposes of carrying on specific activities is referred to as a fund.

Go to **Cram101.com** for the Practice Tests for this Chapter.

Chapter 14. The Basics of Capital Budgeting

Chapter 14. The Basics of Capital Budgeting

Investment	Investment refers to spending for the production and accumulation of capital and additions to inventories. In a financial sense, buying an asset with the expectation of making a return.
Operation	A standardized method or technique that is performed repetitively, often on different materials resulting in different finished goods is called an operation.
Market	A market is, as defined in economics, a social arrangement that allows buyers and sellers to discover information and carry out a voluntary exchange of goods or services.
Strategic plan	The formal document that presents the ways and means by which a strategic goal will be achieved is a strategic plan. A long-term flexible plan that does not regulate activities but rather outlines the means to achieve certain results, and provides the means to alter the course of action should the desired ends change.
Trustee	An independent party appointed to represent the bondholders is referred to as a trustee.
Shareholder wealth maximization	Shareholder wealth maximization refers to maximizing the wealth of the firm's shareholders through achieving the highest possible value for the firm in the marketplace. It is the overriding objective of the firm and should influence all decisions.
Shareholder	A shareholder is an individual or company (including a corporation) that legally owns one or more shares of stock in a joined stock company.
Bankruptcy	Bankruptcy is a legally declared inability or impairment of ability of an individual or organization to pay their creditors.
Consideration	Consideration in contract law, a basic requirement for an enforceable agreement under traditional contract principles, defined in this text as legal value, bargained for and given in exchange for an act or promise. In corporation law, cash or property contributed to a corporation in exchange for shares, or a promise to contribute such cash or property.
Variable	A variable is something measured by a number; it is used to analyze what happens to other things when the size of that number changes.
Cash outflow	Cash flowing out of the business from all sources over a period of time is cash outflow.
Revenue	Revenue is a U.S. business term for the amount of money that a company receives from its activities, mostly from sales of products and/or services to customers.
Analyst	Analyst refers to a person or tool with a primary function of information analysis, generally with a more limited, practical and short term set of goals than a researcher.
Accounting income	The accountant's concept of income is generally based upon the realization principle. Financial accounting income may differ from taxable income. Differences are included in a reconciliation of taxable and accounting income on Schedule M-1 of Form 1120.
Income statement	Income statement refers to a financial statement that presents the revenues and expenses and resulting net income or net loss of a company for a specific period of time.
Accounting	A system that collects and processes financial information about an organization and reports that information to decision makers is referred to as accounting.
Expense	In accounting, an expense represents an event in which an asset is used up or a liability is incurred. In terms of the accounting equation, expenses reduce owners' equity.
Ambulatory care	Ambulatory care is any medical care delivered on an outpatient basis. Many medical conditions do not require hospital admission and can be managed without admission to a hospital. Many medical investigations can be performed on an ambulatory basis, including blood tests, X-rays, endoscopy and even biopsy procedures of superficial organs.
Cash flow forecast	Forecast that predicts the cash inflows and outflows in future periods is a cash flow forecast. It is a company's projected cash receipts and disbursements over a set time horizon.

Go to **Cram101.com** for the Practice Tests for this Chapter.

Chapter 14. The Basics of Capital Budgeting

Chapter 14. The Basics of Capital Budgeting

Operating cash flows	Operating cash flows refers to the cash inflows and cash outflows from the general operating activities of the business; one of the three sections in the statement of cash flows.
Terminal value	In finance, the terminal value of a security is the present value at a future point in time of all future cash flows. It is most often used in multi-stage discounted cash flow analysis, and allows for the limitation of cash flow projections to a several-year period.
Liquidation	Liquidation refers to a process whereby the assets of a business are converted to money. The conversion may be coerced by a legal process to pay off the debt of the business, or to satisfy any other business obligation that the business has not voluntarily satisfied.
Salvage value	In accounting, the salvage value of an asset is its remaining value after depreciation. The estimated value of an asset at the end of its useful life.
Termination	The ending of a corporation that occurs only after the winding-up of the corporation's affairs, the liquidation of its assets, and the distribution of the proceeds to the claimants are referred to as a termination.
Consultant	A professional that provides expert advice in a particular field or area in which customers occassionaly require this type of knowledge is a consultant.
Marketing	Promoting and selling products or services to customers, or prospective customers, is referred to as marketing.
Sunk cost	Sunk cost refers to a cost that has been incurred and cannot be recovered to any significant degree.
Opportunity cost	The cost of something in terms of opportunity foregone. The opportunity cost to a country of producing a unit more of a good, such as for export or to replace an import, is the quantity of some other good that could have been produced instead.
Property	Assets defined in the broadest legal sense. Property includes the unrealized receivables of a cash basis taxpayer, but not services rendered.
Ambulatory surgery	Surgery done in the doctor's office or at a surgical center, and not requiring an overnight stay. Ambulatory surgery is general planned ahead of time. Maybe referred to as one-day, in-and-out, or outpatient surgery.
Market value	Market value refers to the price of an asset agreed on between a willing buyer and a willing seller; the price an asset could demand if it is sold on the open market.
Accounts receivable	Accounts receivable is one of a series of accounting transactions dealing with the billing of customers which owe money to a person, company or organization for goods and services that have been provided to the customer. This is typically done in a one person organization by writing an invoice and mailing or delivering it to each customer.
Working capital	The dollar difference between total current assets and total current liabilities is called working capital.
Inventory	Tangible property held for sale in the normal course of business or used in producing goods or services for sale is an inventory.
Current asset	A current asset is an asset on the balance sheet which is expected to be sold or otherwise used up in the near future, usually within one year.
Current liability	Current liability refers to a debt that can reasonably be expected to be paid from existing current assets or through the creation of other current liabilities, within one year or the operating cycle, whichever is longer.
Liability	A liability is a present obligation of the enterprise arizing from past events, the settlement of which is expected to result in an outflow from the enterprise of resources

Chapter 14. The Basics of Capital Budgeting

Chapter 14. The Basics of Capital Budgeting

	embodying economic benefits.
Inflation	An increase in the overall price level of an economy, usually as measured by the CPI or by the implicit price deflator is called inflation.
Discount	The difference between the face value of a bond and its selling price, when a bond is sold for less than its face value it's referred to as a discount.
Discount rate	Discount rate refers to the rate, per year, at which future values are diminished to make them comparable to values in the present. Can be either subjective or objective.
Inflation rate	The percentage increase in the price level per year is an inflation rate. Alternatively, the inflation rate is the rate of decrease in the purchasing power of money.
Depreciation	Depreciation is an accounting and finance term for the method of attributing the cost of an asset across the useful life of the asset. Depreciation is a reduction in the value of a currency in floating exchange rate.
Complexity	The technical sophistication of the product and hence the amount of understanding required to use it is referred to as complexity. It is the opposite of simplicity.
Preparation	Preparation refers to usually the first stage in the creative process. It includes education and formal training.
Supply	Supply is the aggregate amount of any material good that can be called into being at a certain price point; it comprises one half of the equation of supply and demand. In classical economic theory, a curve representing supply is one of the factors that produce price.
Allowance	Reduction in the selling price of goods extended to the buyer because the goods are defective or of lower quality than the buyer ordered and to encourage a buyer to keep merchandise that would otherwise be returned is the allowance.
Bad debt	In accounting and finance, bad debt is the portion of receivables that can no longer be collected, typically from accounts receivable or loans. Bad debt in accounting is considered an expense.
Overhead cost	An expenses of operating a business over and above the direct costs of producing a product is an overhead cost. They can include utilities (eg, electricity, telephone), advertizing and marketing, and any other costs not billed directly to the client or included in the price of the product.
Assessment	Collecting information and providing feedback to employees about their behavior, communication style, or skills is an assessment.
Evaluation	The consumer's appraisal of the product or brand on important attributes is called evaluation.
Balance	In banking and accountancy, the outstanding balance is the amount of money owned, (or due), that remains in a deposit account (or a loan account) at a given date, after all past remittances, payments and withdrawal have been accounted for. It can be positive (then, in the balance sheet of a firm, it is an asset) or negative (a liability).
Gain	In finance, gain is a profit or an increase in value of an investment such as a stock or bond. Gain is calculated by fair market value or the proceeds from the sale of the investment minus the sum of the purchase price and all costs associated with it.
Labor	People's physical and mental talents and efforts that are used to help produce goods and services are called labor.
Depreciation expense	Depreciation expense refers to the amount recognized as an expense in one period resulting from the periodic recognition of the used portion of the cost of a long-term tangible asset

Chapter 14. The Basics of Capital Budgeting

Chapter 14. The Basics of Capital Budgeting

	over its life.
Amortize	To provide for the payment of a debt by creating a sinking fund or paying in installments is to amortize.
Exempt	Employees who are not covered by the Fair Labor Standards Act are exempt. Exempt employees are not eligible for overtime pay.
Operating expense	In throughput accounting, the cost accounting aspect of Theory of Constraints (TOC), operating expense is the money spent turning inventory into throughput. In TOC, operating expense is limited to costs that vary strictly with the quantity produced, like raw materials and purchased components.
Operating income	Total revenues from operation minus cost of goods sold and operating costs are called operating income.
Cash inflow	Cash coming into the company as the result of a previous investment is a cash inflow.
Debt financing	Obtaining financing by borrowing money is debt financing.
Equity	Equity is the name given to the set of legal principles, in countries following the English common law tradition, which supplement strict rules of law where their application would operate harshly, so as to achieve what is sometimes referred to as "natural justice."
Cost of equity	In finance, the cost of equity is the minimum rate of return a firm must offer shareholders to compensate for waiting for their returns, and for bearing some risk.
Equity capital	Equity capital refers to money raized from within the firm or through the sale of ownership in the firm.
Interest	In finance and economics, interest is the price paid by a borrower for the use of a lender's money. In other words, interest is the amount of paid to "rent" money for a period of time.
Interest expense	The cost a business incurs to borrow money. With respect to bonds payable, the interest expense is calculated by multiplying the market rate of interest by the carrying value of the bonds on the date of the payment.
Cost of debt	The cost of debt is the cost of borrowing money (usually denoted by Kd). It is derived by dividing debt's interest payments on the total market value of the debts.
Modified accelerated cost recovery system	A method in which the cost of tangible property is recovered over a prescribed period of time is the modified accelerated cost recovery system. Enacted by the Economic Recovery Tax Act of 1981 and substantially modified by the Tax Reform Act of 1986, the approach disregards salvage value.
Accelerated Cost Recovery System	Accelerated cost recovery system refers to an accounting depreciation method where the cost of tangible property is weighted more toward the early years of an asset's life.
Recovery	Characterized by rizing output, falling unemployment, rizing profits, and increasing economic activity following a decline is a recovery.
Marginal tax rate	The percentage of an additional dollar of earnings that goes to taxes is referred to as the marginal tax rate.
Book value	The book value of an asset or group of assets is sometimes the price at which they were originally acquired, in many cases equal to purchase price.
Profit	Profit refers to the return to the resource entrepreneurial ability; total revenue minus total cost.
Accounting	Total revenue minus total explicit cost is an accounting profit.

Go to Cram101.com for the Practice Tests for this Chapter.

Chapter 14. The Basics of Capital Budgeting

Chapter 14. The Basics of Capital Budgeting

profit	
Payback period	The amount of time required for a project's after-tax cash inflows to accumulate to an amount that covers the initial investment is a payback period.
Payback	A value that indicates the time period required to recoup an initial investment is a payback. The payback does not include the time-value-of-money concept.
Financial perspective	Financial perspective is one of the four standard perspectives used with the Balanced Scorecard. Financial perspective measures inform an organization whether strategy execution, which is detailed through measures in the other three perspectives, is leading to improved bottom line results.
Return on investment	Return on investment refers to the return a businessperson gets on the money he and other owners invest in the firm; for example, a business that earned $100 on a $1,000 investment would have a ROI of 10 percent: 100 divided by 1000.
Rate of return	A rate of return is a comparison of the money earned (or lost) on an investment to the amount of money invested.
Management	Management characterizes the process of leading and directing all or part of an organization, often a business, through the deployment and manipulation of resources. Early twentieth-century management writer Mary Parker Follett defined management as "the art of getting things done through people."
Dividend	Amount of corporate profits paid out for each share of stock is referred to as dividend.
Required rate of return	Required rate of return refers to the rate of return that investors demand from an investment to compensate them for the amount of risk involved.
Present value	The value today of a stream of payments and/or receipts over time in the future and/or the past, converted to the present using an interest rate. If X t is the amount in period t and r the interest rate, then present value at time t=0 is V = ?T /t.
Discounted cash flow	In finance, the discounted cash flow approach describes a method to value a project or an entire company. The DCF methods determine the present value of future cash flows by discounting them using the appropriate cost of capital.
Internal rate of return	Internal rate of return refers to a discounted cash flow method for evaluating capital budgeting projects. The internal rate of return is a discount rate that makes the present value of the cash inflows equal to the present value of the cash outflows.
Stakeholder	A stakeholder is an individual or group with a vested interest in or expectation for organizational performance. Usually stakeholders can either have an effect on or are affected by an organization.
Stockholder	A stockholder is an individual or company (including a corporation) that legally owns one or more shares of stock in a joined stock company. The shareholders are the owners of a corporation. Companies listed at the stock market strive to enhance shareholder value.
Financial measure	A financial measure is often used as a very simple mechanism to describe the performance of a business or investment. Because they are easily calculated they can not only be used to compare year on year results but also to compare and set norms for a particular type of business or investment.
Net present value	Net present value is a standard method in finance of capital budgeting – the planning of long-term investments. Using this method a potential investment project should be undertaken if the present value of all cash inflows minus the present value of all cash outflows (which equals the net present value) is greater than zero.
Equity	Equity investment generally refers to the buying and holding of shares of stock on a stock

Chapter 14. The Basics of Capital Budgeting

Chapter 14. The Basics of Capital Budgeting

investment	market by individuals and funds in anticipation of income from dividends and capital gain as the value of the stock rises.
Industry	A group of firms that produce identical or similar products is an industry. It is also used specifically to refer to an area of economic production focused on manufacturing which involves large amounts of capital investment before any profit can be realized, also called "heavy industry".
Distortion	Distortion refers to any departure from the ideal of perfect competition that interferes with economic agents maximizing social welfare when they maximize their own.
Points	Loan origination fees that may be deductible as interest by a buyer of property. A seller of property who pays points reduces the selling price by the amount of the points paid for the buyer.
Valuation	In finance, valuation is the process of estimating the market value of a financial asset or liability. They can be done on assets (for example, investments in marketable securities such as stocks, options, business enterprises, or intangible assets such as patents and trademarks) or on liabilities (e.g., Bonds issued by a company).
Merger	Merger refers to the combination of two firms into a single firm.
Severance payment	A severance payment is pay and benefits an employee receives when they leave employment at a company. In addition to the employee's remaining regular pay, it may include some of the following: additional payment based on years of service, payment for unused vacation time or sick leave, medical, dental or life insurance.
Personnel	A collective term for all of the employees of an organization. Personnel is also commonly used to refer to the personnel management function or the organizational unit responsible for administering personnel programs.
Wage	The payment for the service of a unit of labor, per unit time. In trade theory, it is the only payment to labor, usually unskilled labor. In empirical work, wage data may exclude other compenzation, which must be added to get the total cost of employment.
Liquidity	Liquidity refers to the capacity to turn assets into cash, or the amount of assets in a portfolio that have that capacity.
Expected rate of return	Expected rate of return refers to the increase in profit a firm anticipates it will obtain by purchasing capital ; expressed as a percentage of the total cost of the investment activity.
Chief financial officer	Chief financial officer refers to executive responsible for overseeing the financial operations of an organization.
Net investment	In economics, net investment refers to an activity of spending which increases the availability of fixed capital goods or means of production. It is the total spending on new fixed investment minus replacement investment, which simply replaces depreciated capital goods.
Utility	Utility refers to the want-satisfying power of a good or service; the satisfaction or pleasure a consumer obtains from the consumption of a good or service.
Production line	A production line is a set of sequential operations established in a factory whereby materials are put through a refining process to produce an end-product that is suitable for onward consumption; or components are assembled to make a finished article.
Production	The creation of finished goods and services using the factors of production: land, labor, capital, entrepreneurship, and knowledge.
Contribution	In business organization law, the cash or property contributed to a business by its owners is referred to as contribution.

Go to **Cram101.com** for the Practice Tests for this Chapter.

Chapter 14. The Basics of Capital Budgeting

Chapter 14. The Basics of Capital Budgeting

Grant	Grant refers to an intergovernmental transfer of funds. Since the New Deal, state and local governments have become increasingly dependent upon federal grants for an almost infinite variety of programs.
Stock option	A stock option is a specific type of option that uses the stock itself as an underlying instrument to determine the option's pay-off and therefore its value.
Value stock	In financial terminology, a stock that appears attractive using the fundamental criteria of stock valuation because of valuable assets, particularly cash and real estate, owned by its company. A stock may be named a value stock if its earnings per share, cash per share or book value is high relative to the stock price
Holder	A person in possession of a document of title or an instrument payable or indorsed to him, his order, or to bearer is a holder.
Option	A contract that gives the purchaser the option to buy or sell the underlying financial instrument at a specified price, called the exercise price or strike price, within a specific period of time.
Stock	In financial terminology, stock is the capital raized by a corporation, through the issuance and sale of shares.
Capital expenditure	A substantial expenditure that is used by a company to acquire or upgrade physical assets such as equipment, property, industrial buildings, including those which improve the quality and life of an asset is referred to as a capital expenditure.
Financial management	The job of managing a firm's resources so it can meet its goals and objectives is called financial management.
Financial manager	Managers who make recommendations to top executives regarding strategies for improving the financial strength of a firm are referred to as a financial manager.
Administration	Administration refers to the management and direction of the affairs of governments and institutions; a collective term for all policymaking officials of a government; the execution and implementation of public policy.
Contribution margin analysis	Contribution margin analysis is a technique used in brand marketing and product management to help a company decide what product(s) to add to its product portfolio. The manager asks what will happen to profits if a new product is added or an existing product is discontinued. Calculations take into account additional revenues, additional costs, effects on other products in the portfolio and competitors' reactions.
Contribution margin	A company's contribution margin can be expressed as the percentage of each sale that remains after the variable costs are subtracted. In simplest terms, the contribution margin is total revenue minus total variable cost.
Case study	A case study is a particular method of qualitative research. Rather than using large samples and following a rigid protocol to examine a limited number of variables, case study methods involve an in-depth, longitudinal examination of a single instance or event: a case. They provide a systematic way of looking at events, collecting data, analyzing information, and reporting the results.
Margin	A deposit by a buyer in stocks with a seller or a stockbroker, as security to cover fluctuations in the market in reference to stocks that the buyer has purchased but for which he has not paid is a margin. Commodities are also traded on margin.
Journal	Book of original entry, in which transactions are recorded in a general ledger system, is referred to as a journal.

Chapter 14. The Basics of Capital Budgeting

Chapter 15. Project Risk Assessment and Incorporation

Assessment	Collecting information and providing feedback to employees about their behavior, communication style, or skills is an assessment.
Project risk assessment	Project risk assessment refers to a method for determining the propensity for a Six-Sigma project to achieve desired results.
Capital budgeting	Capital budgeting is the planning process used to determine a firm's long term investments such as new machinery, replacement machinery, new plants, new products, and research and development projects.
Cash flow	In finance, cash flow refers to the amounts of cash being received and spent by a business during a defined period of time, sometimes tied to a specific project. Most of the time they are being used to determine gaps in the liquid position of a company.
Capital	Capital generally refers to financial wealth, especially that used to start or maintain a business. In classical economics, capital is one of four factors of production, the others being land and labor and entrepreneurship.
Investment	Investment refers to spending for the production and accumulation of capital and additions to inventories. In a financial sense, buying an asset with the expectation of making a return.
Rate of return	A rate of return is a comparison of the money earned (or lost) on an investment to the amount of money invested.
Required rate of return	Required rate of return refers to the rate of return that investors demand from an investment to compensate them for the amount of risk involved.
Cost of capital	Cost of capital refers to the percentage cost of funds used for acquiring resources for an organization, typically a weighted average of the firms cost of equity and cost of debt.
Firm	An organization that employs resources to produce a good or service for profit and owns and operates one or more plants is referred to as a firm.
Discount rate	Discount rate refers to the rate, per year, at which future values are diminished to make them comparable to values in the present. Can be either subjective or objective .
Discount	The difference between the face value of a bond and its selling price, when a bond is sold for less than its face value it's referred to as a discount.
Financial risk	The risk related to the inability of the firm to meet its debt obligations as they come due is called financial risk.
Context	The effect of the background under which a message often takes on more and richer meaning is a context. Context is especially important in cross-cultural interactions because some cultures are said to be high context or low context.
Portfolio effect	Portfolio effect refers to the impact of a given investment on the overall risk-return composition of the firm. A firm must consider not only the individual investment characteristics of a project but also how the project relates to the entire portfolio of undertakings.
Portfolio	In finance, a portfolio is a collection of investments held by an institution or a private individual. Holding but not always a portfolio is part of an investment and risk-limiting strategy called diversification. By owning several assets, certain types of risk (in particular specific risk) can be reduced.
Equity	Equity is the name given to the set of legal principles, in countries following the English common law tradition, which supplement strict rules of law where their application would operate harshly, so as to achieve what is sometimes referred to as "natural justice."
Market risk	Market risk is the risk that the value of an investment will decrease due to moves in market

Chapter 15. Project Risk Assessment and Incorporation

Chapter 15. Project Risk Assessment and Incorporation

factors.

Shareholder	A shareholder is an individual or company (including a corporation) that legally owns one or more shares of stock in a joined stock company.
Market	A market is, as defined in economics, a social arrangement that allows buyers and sellers to discover information and carry out a voluntary exchange of goods or services.
Stock	In financial terminology, stock is the capital raized by a corporation, through the issuance and sale of shares.
Form of ownership	Distinguishes retail outlets based on whether individuals, corporate chains, or contractual systems own the outlet is called form of ownership.
Expected return	Expected return refers to the return on an asset expected over the next period.
Standard deviation	A measure of the spread or dispersion of a series of numbers around the expected value is the standard deviation. The standard deviation tells us how well the expected value represents a series of values.
Net present value	Net present value is a standard method in finance of capital budgeting – the planning of long-term investments. Using this method a potential investment project should be undertaken if the present value of all cash inflows minus the present value of all cash outflows (which equals the net present value) is greater than zero.
Present value	The value today of a stream of payments and/or receipts over time in the future and/or the past, converted to the present using an interest rate. If X_t is the amount in period t and r the interest rate, then present value at time t=0 is V = ?T /t.
Internal rate of return	Internal rate of return refers to a discounted cash flow method for evaluating capital budgeting projects. The internal rate of return is a discount rate that makes the present value of the cash inflows equal to the present value of the cash outflows.
Service	Service refers to a "non tangible product" that is not embodied in a physical good and that typically effects some change in another product, person, or institution. Contrasts with good.
Contribution	In business organization law, the cash or property contributed to a business by its owners is referred to as contribution.
Volatility	Volatility refers to the extent to which an economic variable, such as a price or an exchange rate, moves up and down over time.
Industry	A group of firms that produce identical or similar products is an industry. It is also used specifically to refer to an area of economic production focused on manufacturing which involves large amounts of capital investment before any profit can be realized, also called "heavy industry".
Shareholder wealth maximization	Shareholder wealth maximization refers to maximizing the wealth of the firm's shareholders through achieving the highest possible value for the firm in the marketplace. It is the overriding objective of the firm and should influence all decisions.
Diversified portfolio	Diversified portfolio refers to a portfolio that includes a variety of assets whose prices are not likely all to change together. In international economics, this usually means holding assets denominated in different currencies.
Primary factor	Primary factor refers to an input that exists as a stock, providing services that contribute to production. The stock is not used up in production, although it may deteriorate with use, providing a smaller flow of services later.
Correlation	A correlation is the measure of the extent to which two economic or statistical variables

Chapter 15. Project Risk Assessment and Incorporation

Chapter 15. Project Risk Assessment and Incorporation

	move together, normalized so that its values range from -1 to +1. It is defined as the covariance of the two variables divided by the square root of the product of their variances.
Positively correlated	Positively correlated refers to values or amounts of two items that move in the same direction. In accounting and finance, the amount of risk and the amount of return on an investment move in the same direction.
Proxy	Proxy refers to a person who is authorized to vote the shares of another person. Also, the written authorization empowering a person to vote the shares of another person.
Sensitivity analysis	A what-if technique that managers use to examine how a result will change if the original predicted data are not achieved or if an underlying assumption changes is sensitivity analysis.
Distribution	Distribution in economics, the manner in which total output and income is distributed among individuals or factors.
Variable	A variable is something measured by a number; it is used to analyze what happens to other things when the size of that number changes.
Probability distribution	A specification of the probabilities for each possible value of a random variable is called probability distribution.
Expected value	A representative value from a probability distribution arrived at by multiplying each outcome by the associated probability and summing up the values is called the expected value.
Salvage value	In accounting, the salvage value of an asset is its remaining value after depreciation. The estimated value of an asset at the end of its useful life.
Slope	The slope of a line in the plane containing the x and y axes is generally represented by the letter m, and is defined as the change in the y coordinate divided by the corresponding change in the x coordinate, between two distinct points on the line.
Scenario analysis	Scenario analysis is a process of analyzing possible future events by considering alternative possible outcomes. The analysis is designed to allow improved decision-making by allowing more complete consideration of outcomes and their implications.
Economy	The income, expenditures, and resources that affect the cost of running a business and household are called an economy.
Points	Loan origination fees that may be deductible as interest by a buyer of property. A seller of property who pays points reduces the selling price by the amount of the points paid for the buyer.
Utility	Utility refers to the want-satisfying power of a good or service; the satisfaction or pleasure a consumer obtains from the consumption of a good or service.
Cash outflow	Cash flowing out of the business from all sources over a period of time is cash outflow.
Opportunity cost	The cost of something in terms of opportunity foregone. The opportunity cost to a country of producing a unit more of a good, such as for export or to replace an import, is the quantity of some other good that could have been produced instead.
Valuation	In finance, valuation is the process of estimating the market value of a financial asset or liability. They can be done on assets (for example, investments in marketable securities such as stocks, options, business enterprises, or intangible assets such as patents and trademarks) or on liabilities (e.g., Bonds issued by a company).
Risk premium	In finance, the risk premium can be the expected rate of return above the risk-free interest rate.
Premium	Premium refers to the fee charged by an insurance company for an insurance policy. The rate

Go to **Cram101.com** for the Practice Tests for this Chapter.

Chapter 15. Project Risk Assessment and Incorporation

Chapter 15. Project Risk Assessment and Incorporation

	of losses must be relatively predictable: In order to set the premium (prices) insurers must be able to estimate them accurately.
Interest	In finance and economics, interest is the price paid by a borrower for the use of a lender's money. In other words, interest is the amount of paid to "rent" money for a period of time.
Allocate	Allocate refers to the assignment of income for various tax purposes. A multistate corporation's nonbusiness income usually is distributed to the state where the nonbusiness assets are located; it is not apportioned with the rest of the entity's income.
Revenue	Revenue is a U.S. business term for the amount of money that a company receives from its activities, mostly from sales of products and/or services to customers.
Consideration	Consideration in contract law, a basic requirement for an enforceable agreement under traditional contract principles, defined in this text as legal value, bargained for and given in exchange for an act or promise. In corporation law, cash or property contributed to a corporation in exchange for shares, or a promise to contribute such cash or property.
Contract	A contract is a "promise" or an "agreement" that is enforced or recognized by the law. In the civil law, a contract is considered to be part of the general law of obligations.
Bid	A bid price is a price offered by a buyer when he/she buys a good. In the context of stock trading on a stock exchange, the bid price is the highest price a buyer of a stock is willing to pay for a share of that given stock.
Profit	Profit refers to the return to the resource entrepreneurial ability; total revenue minus total cost.
Market value	Market value refers to the price of an asset agreed on between a willing buyer and a willing seller; the price an asset could demand if it is sold on the open market.
Subsidiary	A company that is controlled by another company or corporation is a subsidiary.
Capital structure	Capital Structure refers to the way a corporation finances itself through some combination of equity sales, equity options, bonds, and loans. Optimal capital structure refers to the particular combination that minimizes the cost of capital while maximizing the stock price.
Business risk	The risk related to the inability of the firm to hold its competitive position and maintain stability and growth in earnings is business risk.
Estate	An estate is the totality of the legal rights, interests, entitlements and obligations attaching to property. In the context of wills and probate, it refers to the totality of the property which the deceased owned or in which some interest was held.
Asset	An item of property, such as land, capital, money, a share in ownership, or a claim on others for future payment, such as a bond or a bank deposit is an asset.
Capital budget	A long-term budget that shows planned acquisition and disposal of capital assets, such as land, building, and equipment is a capital budget. Also a separate budget used by state governments for items such as new construction, major renovations, and acquisition of physical property.
Budget	Budget refers to an account, usually for a year, of the planned expenditures and the expected receipts of an entity. For a government, the receipts are tax revenues.
Chief financial officer	Chief financial officer refers to executive responsible for overseeing the financial operations of an organization.
Categorizing	The act of placing strengths and weaknesses into categories in generic internal assessment is called categorizing.
Capital	The capital requirement is a bank regulation, which sets a framework on how banks and

Chapter 15. Project Risk Assessment and Incorporation

Chapter 15. Project Risk Assessment and Incorporation

requirement	depository institutions must handle their capital. The categorization of assets and capital is highly standardized so that it can be risk weighted.
Mistake	In contract law a mistake is incorrect understanding by one or more parties to a contract and may be used as grounds to invalidate the agreement. Common law has identified three different types of mistake in contract: unilateral mistake, mutual mistake, and common mistake.
Capital rationing	Capital rationing occurs when a corporation has more dollars of capital budgeting projects with positive net present values than it has money to invest in them. Therefore, some projects that should be accepted are excluded because financial capital is rationed.
Rationing	Rationing is the controlled distribution of resources and scarce goods or services: it restricts how much people are allowed to buy or consume.
Fund	Independent accounting entity with a self-balancing set of accounts segregated for the purposes of carrying on specific activities is referred to as a fund.
Financial perspective	Financial perspective is one of the four standard perspectives used with the Balanced Scorecard. Financial perspective measures inform an organization whether strategy execution, which is detailed through measures in the other three perspectives, is leading to improved bottom line results.
Diversification	Investing in a collection of assets whose returns do not always move together, with the result that overall risk is lower than for individual assets is referred to as diversification.
Stockholder	A stockholder is an individual or company (including a corporation) that legally owns one or more shares of stock in a joined stock company. The shareholders are the owners of a corporation. Companies listed at the stock market strive to enhance shareholder value.
Stakeholder	A stakeholder is an individual or group with a vested interest in or expectation for organizational performance. Usually stakeholders can either have an effect on or are affected by an organization.
Decision tree	In decision theory, a decision tree is a graph of decisions and their possible consequences, (including resource costs and risks) used to create a plan to reach a goal.
Management	Management characterizes the process of leading and directing all or part of an organization, often a business, through the deployment and manipulation of resources. Early twentieth-century management writer Mary Parker Follett defined management as "the art of getting things done through people."
Debt financing	Obtaining financing by borrowing money is debt financing.
Profitability index	The present value of a project's future cash flows, divided by the initial investment is referred to as the profitability index.
Cash inflow	Cash coming into the company as the result of a previous investment is a cash inflow.
Acquisition	A company's purchase of the property and obligations of another company is an acquisition.
Technology	The body of knowledge and techniques that can be used to combine economic resources to produce goods and services is called technology.
Financial management	The job of managing a firm's resources so it can meet its goals and objectives is called financial management.
Evaluation	The consumer's appraisal of the product or brand on important attributes is called evaluation.
Practical approach	The approach to decision-making that combines the steps of the rational approach with the conditions in the behavioral approach to create a more realistic process for making decisions

Go to **Cram101.com** for the Practice Tests for this Chapter.

Chapter 15. Project Risk Assessment and Incorporation

Chapter 15. Project Risk Assessment and Incorporation

in organizations is referred to as practical approach.

Administration	Administration refers to the management and direction of the affairs of governments and institutions; a collective term for all policymaking officials of a government; the execution and implementation of public policy.
Harvard Business Review	Harvard Business Review is a research-based magazine written for business practitioners, it claims a high ranking business readership and enjoys the reverence of academics, executives, and management consultants. It has been the frequent publishing home for well known scholars and management thinkers.
Journal	Book of original entry, in which transactions are recorded in a general ledger system, is referred to as a journal.
Capital expenditure	A substantial expenditure that is used by a company to acquire or upgrade physical assets such as equipment, property, industrial buildings, including those which improve the quality and life of an asset is referred to as a capital expenditure.

Chapter 15. Project Risk Assessment and Incorporation

Chapter 16. Current Asset Management and Financing

Security	Security refers to a claim on the borrower future income that is sold by the borrower to the lender. A security is a type of transferable interest representing financial value.
Marketable securities	Marketable securities refer to securities that are readily traded in the secondary securities market.
Inventory management	The planning, coordinating, and controlling activities related to the flow of inventory into, through, and out of an organization is referred to as inventory management.
Management	Management characterizes the process of leading and directing all or part of an organization, often a business, through the deployment and manipulation of resources. Early twentieth-century management writer Mary Parker Follett defined management as "the art of getting things done through people."
Inventory	Tangible property held for sale in the normal course of business or used in producing goods or services for sale is an inventory.
Financial management	The job of managing a firm's resources so it can meet its goals and objectives is called financial management.
Current asset	A current asset is an asset on the balance sheet which is expected to be sold or otherwise used up in the near future, usually within one year.
Asset	An item of property, such as land, capital, money, a share in ownership, or a claim on others for future payment, such as a bond or a bank deposit is an asset.
Brief	Brief refers to a statement of a party's case or legal arguments, usually prepared by an attorney. Also used to make legal arguments before appellate courts.
Current liability	Current liability refers to a debt that can reasonably be expected to be paid from existing current assets or through the creation of other current liabilities, within one year or the operating cycle, whichever is longer.
Liability	A liability is a present obligation of the enterprise arizing from past events, the settlement of which is expected to result in an outflow from the enterprise of resources embodying economic benefits.
Operation	A standardized method or technique that is performed repetitively, often on different materials resulting in different finished goods is called an operation.
Ambulatory care	Ambulatory care is any medical care delivered on an outpatient basis. Many medical conditions do not require hospital admission and can be managed without admission to a hospital. Many medical investigations can be performed on an ambulatory basis, including blood tests, X-rays, endoscopy and even biopsy procedures of superficial organs.
Service	Service refers to a "non tangible product" that is not embodied in a physical good and that typically effects some change in another product, person, or institution. Contrasts with good.
Peak	Peak refers to the point in the business cycle when an economic expansion reaches its highest point before turning down. Contrasts with trough.
Accounts receivable	Accounts receivable is one of a series of accounting transactions dealing with the billing of customers which owe money to a person, company or organization for goods and services that have been provided to the customer. This is typically done in a one person organization by writing an invoice and mailing or delivering it to each customer.
Preparation	Preparation refers to usually the first stage in the creative process. It includes education and formal training.
Accounts payable	A written record of all vendors to whom the business firm owes money is referred to as

Chapter 16. Current Asset Management and Financing

Chapter 16. Current Asset Management and Financing

	accounts payable.
Accrual	An accrual is an accounting event in which the transaction is recognized when the action takes place, instead of when cash is disbursed or received.
Balance sheet	A statement of the assets, liabilities, and net worth of a firm or individual at some given time often at the end of its "fiscal year," is referred to as a balance sheet.
Capital	Capital generally refers to financial wealth, especially that used to start or maintain a business. In classical economics, capital is one of four factors of production, the others being land and labor and entrepreneurship.
Balance	In banking and accountancy, the outstanding balance is the amount of money owned, (or due), that remains in a deposit account (or a loan account) at a given date, after all past remittances, payments and withdrawal have been accounted for. It can be positive (then, in the balance sheet of a firm, it is an asset) or negative (a liability).
Equity	Equity is the name given to the set of legal principles, in countries following the English common law tradition, which supplement strict rules of law where their application would operate harshly, so as to achieve what is sometimes referred to as "natural justice."
Firm	An organization that employs resources to produce a good or service for profit and owns and operates one or more plants is referred to as a firm.
Notes payable	Notes payable refers to an obligation in the form of a written promissory note. It is a balance sheet term referring to a company's outstanding bank loans.
Business cycle	Business cycle refers to the pattern followed by macroeconomic variables, such as GDP and unemployment that rise and fall irregularly over time, relative to trend.
Recession	A significant decline in economic activity. In the U.S., recession is approximately defined as two successive quarters of falling GDP, as judged by NBER.
Contract	A contract is a "promise" or an "agreement" that is enforced or recognized by the law. In the civil law, a contract is considered to be part of the general law of obligations.
Investment	Investment refers to spending for the production and accumulation of capital and additions to inventories. In a financial sense, buying an asset with the expectation of making a return.
Policy	Similar to a script in that a policy can be a less than completely rational decision-making method. Involves the use of a pre-existing set of decision steps for any problem that presents itself.
Slope	The slope of a line in the plane containing the x and y axes is generally represented by the letter m, and is defined as the change in the y coordinate divided by the corresponding change in the x coordinate, between two distinct points on the line.
Credit	Credit refers to a recording as positive in the balance of payments, any transaction that gives rise to a payment into the country, such as an export, the sale of an asset, or borrowing from abroad.
Profit	Profit refers to the return to the resource entrepreneurial ability; total revenue minus total cost.
Holding	The holding is a court's determination of a matter of law based on the issue presented in the particular case. In other words: under this law, with these facts, this result.
Labor	People's physical and mental talents and efforts that are used to help produce goods and services are called labor.
Safety stock	Safety stock is additional inventory planned to buffer against the variability in supply and demand plans, that could otherwise result in inventory shortages.

Chapter 16. Current Asset Management and Financing

Chapter 16. Current Asset Management and Financing

Realization	Realization is the sale of assets when an entity is being liquidated.
Stock	In financial terminology, stock is the capital raized by a corporation, through the issuance and sale of shares.
Expected return	Expected return refers to the return on an asset expected over the next period.
Converse	Converse is an American shoe company which has been making shoes since the early 20th century. The company's main turning point came in 1917 when the Converse All-Star basketball shoe was introduced. This was a real innovation at the time, considering the sport was only 25 years old.
Business risk	The risk related to the inability of the firm to hold its competitive position and maintain stability and growth in earnings is business risk.
Fixed asset	Fixed asset, also known as property, plant, and equipment (PP&E), is a term used in accountancy for assets and property which cannot easily be converted into cash. This can be compared with current assets such as cash or bank accounts, which are described as liquid assets. In most cases, only tangible assets are referred to as fixed.
Permanent current assets	Permanent current assets refer to current assets that will not be reduced or converted to cash within the normal operating cycle of the firm. Though from a strict accounting standpoint the assets should be removed from the current assets category, they generally are
Temporary current assets	Current assets that will be reduced or converted to cash within the normal operating cycle of the firm are referred to as temporary current assets. That portion of a firm`s current assets that fluctuates in response to seasonal or anticipated short-term.
Accounting	A system that collects and processes financial information about an organization and reports that information to decision makers is referred to as accounting.
Depreciation	Depreciation is an accounting and finance term for the method of attributing the cost of an asset across the useful life of the asset. Depreciation is a reduction in the value of a currency in floating exchange rate.
Cash flow	In finance, cash flow refers to the amounts of cash being received and spent by a business during a defined period of time, sometimes tied to a specific project. Most of the time they are being used to determine gaps in the liquid position of a company.
Interest rate	The rate of return on bonds, loans, or deposits. When one speaks of 'the' interest rate, it is usually in a model where there is only one.
Interest	In finance and economics, interest is the price paid by a borrower for the use of a lender's money. In other words, interest is the amount of paid to "rent" money for a period of time.
Lender	Suppliers and financial institutions that lend money to companies is referred to as a lender.
Liquidity	Liquidity refers to the capacity to turn assets into cash, or the amount of assets in a portfolio that have that capacity.
Matching	Matching refers to an accounting concept that establishes when expenses are recognized. Expenses are matched with the revenues they helped to generate and are recognized when those revenues are recognized.
Maturity	Maturity refers to the final payment date of a loan or other financial instrument, after which point no further interest or principal need be paid.
Financial risk	The risk related to the inability of the firm to meet its debt obligations as they come due is called financial risk.
Acceleration	Acceleration refers to the shortening of the time for the performance of a contract or the payment of a note by the operation of some provision in the contract or note itself.

Go to **Cram101.com** for the Practice Tests for this Chapter.

Chapter 16. Current Asset Management and Financing

Chapter 16. Current Asset Management and Financing

Fund	Independent accounting entity with a self-balancing set of accounts segregated for the purposes of carrying on specific activities is referred to as a fund.
Lockbox system	Lockbox system refers to a procedure used to expedite cash inflows to a business. Customers are requested to forward their checks to a post office box in their geographic region, and a local bank picks up the checks and processes them for rapid collection. Funds are then wired to the corporate home office for immediate use.
Points	Loan origination fees that may be deductible as interest by a buyer of property. A seller of property who pays points reduces the selling price by the amount of the points paid for the buyer.
Economies of scale	In economics, returns to scale and economies of scale are related terms that describe what happens as the scale of production increases. They are different terms and not to be used interchangeably.
Economy	The income, expenditures, and resources that affect the cost of running a business and household are called an economy.
Financial institution	A financial institution acts as an agent that provides financial services for its clients. Financial institutions generally fall under financial regulation from a government authority.
Automated clearinghouse	Automated clearinghouse transfers information between one financial institution and another and from account to account via computer tape. There are approximately 30 regional clearinghouses throughout the United States that claim the membership of over 10,000 financial institutions.
Controlling	A management function that involves determining whether or not an organization is progressing toward its goals and objectives, and taking corrective action if it is not is called controlling.
Centralization	A structural policy in which decision-making authority is concentrated at the top of the organizational hierarchy is referred to as centralization.
Payables	Obligations to make future economic sacrifices, usually cash payments, are referred to as payables. Same as current liabilities.
Line of credit	Line of credit refers to a given amount of unsecured short-term funds a bank will lend to a business, provided the funds are readily available.
Portfolio	In finance, a portfolio is a collection of investments held by an institution or a private individual. Holding but not always a portfolio is part of an investment and risk-limiting strategy called diversification. By owning several assets, certain types of risk (in particular specific risk) can be reduced.
Marginal cost	Marginal cost refers to the increase in cost that accompanies a unit increase in output; the partial derivative of the cost function with respect to output.
Expense	In accounting, an expense represents an event in which an asset is used up or a liability is incurred. In terms of the accounting equation, expenses reduce owners' equity.
Personnel	A collective term for all of the employees of an organization. Personnel is also commonly used to refer to the personnel management function or the organizational unit responsible for administering personnel programs.
Business operations	Business operations are those activities involved in the running of a business for the purpose of producing value for the stakeholders. The outcome of business operations is the harvesting of value from assets owned by a business.
Marketing	Promoting and selling products or services to customers, or prospective customers, is referred to as marketing.

Go to **Cram101.com** for the Practice Tests for this Chapter.

Chapter 16. Current Asset Management and Financing

Chapter 16. Current Asset Management and Financing

Management system	A management system is the framework of processes and procedures used to ensure that an organization can fulfill all tasks required to achieve its objectives.
Commercial paper	Commercial paper is a money market security issued by large banks and corporations. It is generally not used to finance long-term investments but rather for purchases of inventory or to manage working capital. It is commonly bought by money funds (the issuing amounts are often too high for individual investors), and is generally regarded as a very safe investment.
Treasury bills	Short-term obligations of the federal government are treasury bills. They are like zero coupon bonds in that they do not pay interest prior to maturity; instead they are sold at a discount of the par value to create a positive yield to maturity.
Negotiable	A negotiable instrument is one that can be bought and sold after being issued - in other words, it is a tradable instrument.
Certificates of deposit	Certificates of deposit refer to a certificate offered by banks, savings and loans, and other financial institutions for the deposit of funds at a given interest rate over a specified time period.
Preferred stock	Stock that has specified rights over common stock is a preferred stock.
Dividend	Amount of corporate profits paid out for each share of stock is referred to as dividend.
Mutual fund	A mutual fund is a form of collective investment that pools money from many investors and invests the money in stocks, bonds, short-term money market instruments, and/or other securities. In a mutual fund, the fund manager trades the fund's underlying securities, realizing capital gains or loss, and collects the dividend or interest income.
Direct investment	Direct investment refers to a domestic firm actually investing in and owning a foreign subsidiary or division.
Net income	Net income is equal to the income that a firm has after subtracting costs and expenses from the total revenue. Expenses will typically include tax expense.
Pension fund	Amounts of money put aside by corporations, nonprofit organizations, or unions to cover part of the financial needs of members when they retire is a pension fund.
Pension	A pension is a steady income given to a person (usually after retirement). Pensions are typically payments made in the form of a guaranteed annuity to a retired or disabled employee.
Endowment	Endowment refers to the amount of something that a person or country simply has, rather than their having somehow to acquire it.
Foundation	A Foundation is a type of philanthropic organization set up by either individuals or institutions as a legal entity (either as a corporation or trust) with the purpose of distributing grants to support causes in line with the goals of the foundation.
Investment portfolio	An investment portfolio is an aggregate of investments, such as stocks, bonds, real estate, arts or even fine wines. What distinguishes an investment portfolio from net worth is that some asset classes are not considered investments.
Industry	A group of firms that produce identical or similar products is an industry. It is also used specifically to refer to an area of economic production focused on manufacturing which involves large amounts of capital investment before any profit can be realized, also called "heavy industry".
Credit sale	A credit sale occurs when a customer does not pay cash at the time of the sale but instead agrees to pay later. The sale occurs now, with payment from the customer to follow at a later time.

Go to **Cram101.com** for the Practice Tests for this Chapter.

Chapter 16. Current Asset Management and Financing

Chapter 16. Current Asset Management and Financing

Accumulation	The acquisition of an increasing quantity of something. The accumulation of factors, especially capital, is a primary mechanism for economic growth.
Average collection period	The average amount of time that a receivable is outstanding, calculated by dividing 365 days by the receivables turnover ratio is an average collection period.
Revenue	Revenue is a U.S. business term for the amount of money that a company receives from its activities, mostly from sales of products and/or services to customers.
Carrying costs	Carrying costs refers to costs that arise while holding an inventory of goods for sale.
Carrying cost	The cost to hold an asset, usually inventory is called a carrying cost. For inventory, a carrying cost includes such items as interest, warehousing costs, insurance, and material-handling expenses.
Complexity	The technical sophistication of the product and hence the amount of understanding required to use it is referred to as complexity. It is the opposite of simplicity.
Trend	Trend refers to the long-term movement of an economic variable, such as its average rate of increase or decrease over enough years to encompass several business cycles.
Verification	Verification refers to the final stage of the creative process where the validity or truthfulness of the insight is determined. The feedback portion of communication in which the receiver sends a message to the source indicating receipt of the message and the degree to which he or she understood the message.
Insurance	Insurance refers to a system by which individuals can reduce their exposure to risk of large losses by spreading the risks among a large number of persons.
Intervention	Intervention refers to an activity in which a government buys or sells its currency in the foreign exchange market in order to affect its currency's exchange rate.
Electronic data interchange	Electronic data interchange refers to the direct exchange between organizations of data via a computer-to-computer interface.
Exchange	The trade of things of value between buyer and seller so that each is better off after the trade is called the exchange.
Supply chain	Supply chain refers to the flow of goods, services, and information from the initial sources of materials and services to the delivery of products to consumers.
Supply	Supply is the aggregate amount of any material good that can be called into being at a certain price point; it comprises one half of the equation of supply and demand. In classical economic theory, a curve representing supply is one of the factors that produce price.
Supply chain management	Supply chain management deals with the planning and execution issues involved in managing a supply chain. Supply chain management spans all movement and storage of raw materials, work-in-process inventory, and finished goods from point-of-origin to point-of-consumption.
Purchasing	Purchasing refers to the function in a firm that searches for quality material resources, finds the best suppliers, and negotiates the best price for goods and services.
Inventory control	Inventory control, in the field of loss prevention, are systems designed to introduce technical barriers to shoplifting.
Control system	A control system is a device or set of devices that manage the behavior of other devices. Some devices or systems are not controllable. A control system is an interconnection of components connected or related in such a manner as to command, direct, or regulate itself or another system.
Usage rate	Usage rate refers to quantity consumed or patronage-store visits during a specific period;

Chapter 16. Current Asset Management and Financing

Chapter 16. Current Asset Management and Financing

	varies significantly among different customer groups.
Control process	A process involving gathering processed data, analyzing processed data, and using this information to make adjustments to the process is a control process.
Warehouse	Warehouse refers to a location, often decentralized, that a firm uses to store, consolidate, age, or mix stock; house product-recall programs; or ease tax burdens.
Materials management	Materials management refers to the activity that controls the transmission of physical materials through the value chain, from procurement through production and into distribution.
Bond indenture	Bond contract that specifies the stated rate of interest and the face value of the bond as well as other contractual provisions is called the bond indenture. A company's bond indenture will cover all bonds issued by that company and also list all bond covenants.
Credit market	A credit market is where borrowers come together with lenders to determine conditions of exchange such as interest rates and the duration of a loan.
Indenture	A bond contract that specifies the legal provisions of a bond issue is called an indenture.
Market	A market is, as defined in economics, a social arrangement that allows buyers and sellers to discover information and carry out a voluntary exchange of goods or services.
Bond	Bond refers to a debt instrument, issued by a borrower and promising a specified stream of payments to the purchaser, usually regular interest payments plus a final repayment of principal.
Restrictive covenant	A restrictive covenant is a legal obligation imposed in a deed by the seller upon the buyer of real estate to do or not to do something.
Covenant	A covenant is a signed written agreement between two or more parties. Also referred to as a contract.
Yield curve	In finance, the yield curve is the relation between the interest rate (or cost of borrowing) and the maturity of the debt for a given borrower in a given currency.
Yield	The interest rate that equates a future value or an annuity to a given present value is a yield.
Financing statement	A document, usually a multicopy form, filed in a public office serving as constructive notice to the world that a creditor claims a security interest in collateral that belongs to a certain named debtor is a financing statement.
Wage	The payment for the service of a unit of labor, per unit time. In trade theory, it is the only payment to labor, usually unskilled labor. In empirical work, wage data may exclude other compenzation, which must be added to get the total cost of employment.
Trade credit	Trade credit refers to an amount that is loaned to an exporter to be repaid when the exports are paid for by the foreign importer.
Discount	The difference between the face value of a bond and its selling price, when a bond is sold for less than its face value it's referred to as a discount.
Free trade	Free trade refers to a situation in which there are no artificial barriers to trade, such as tariffs and quotas. Usually used, often only implicitly, with frictionless trade, so that it implies that there are no barriers to trade of any kind.
Terms of trade	Terms of trade refers to the rate at which units of one product can be exchanged for units of another product; the price of a good or service; the amount of one good or service that must be given up to obtain 1 unit of another good or service.
Commercial bank	A firm that engages in the business of banking is a commercial bank.

Chapter 16. Current Asset Management and Financing

Chapter 16. Current Asset Management and Financing

Promissory note	Commercial paper or instrument in which the maker promises to pay a specific sum of money to another person, to his order, or to bearer is referred to as a promissory note.
Compensating balance	A required minimum amount of funds that a firm receiving a loan must keep in a checking account at the lending bank is called compensating balance.
Stated interest rate	Rate of interest specified in the bond contract that will be paid at specified intervals over the life of the bond is the stated interest rate.
Interest expense	The cost a business incurs to borrow money. With respect to bonds payable, the interest expense is calculated by multiplying the market rate of interest by the carrying value of the bonds on the date of the payment.
Revolving credit agreement	A line of credit that is guaranteed by the bank is called a revolving credit agreement.
Prime rate	The rate that a bank charges its most creditworthy customers is referred to as the prime rate.
Administrative cost	An administrative cost is all executive, organizational, and clerical costs associated with the general management of an organization rather than with manufacturing, marketing, or selling
Secured loan	Secured loan refers to a loan backed by something valuable, such as property.
Collateral	Property that is pledged to the lender to guarantee payment in the event that the borrower is unable to make debt payments is called collateral.
Real property	Real property is a legal term encompassing real estate and ownership interests in real estate (immovable property).
Property	Assets defined in the broadest legal sense. Property includes the unrealized receivables of a cash basis taxpayer, but not services rendered.
Face value	The nominal or par value of an instrument as expressed on its face is referred to as the face value.
Factoring	In mathematics, factorization or factoring is the decomposition of an object into a product of other objects, or factors, which when multiplied together give the original.
Buyer	A buyer refers to a role in the buying center with formal authority and responsibility to select the supplier and negotiate the terms of the contract.
Default	In finance, default occurs when a debtor has not met its legal obligations according to the debt contract, e.g. it has not made a scheduled payment, or violated a covenant (condition) of the debt contract.
Unsecured loan	A loan that's not backed by any specific assets is an unsecured loan. The risk of repossession does not exist. This doesn't mean that the lender cannot take legal action in order to recover his money. However, such a legal process would be significantly longer and more expensive than with secured loans.
Credit risk	The risk of loss due to a counterparty defaulting on a contract, or more generally the risk of loss due to some "credit event" is called credit risk.
Consideration	Consideration in contract law, a basic requirement for an enforceable agreement under traditional contract principles, defined in this text as legal value, bargained for and given in exchange for an act or promise. In corporation law, cash or property contributed to a corporation in exchange for shares, or a promise to contribute such cash or property.
Bad debt	In accounting and finance, bad debt is the portion of receivables that can no longer be

Chapter 16. Current Asset Management and Financing

Chapter 16. Current Asset Management and Financing

	collected, typically from accounts receivable or loans. Bad debt in accounting is considered an expense.
Principal	In agency law, one under whose direction an agent acts and for whose benefit that agent acts is a principal.
Compensating balances	Compensating balances refer to a bank requirement that business customers maintain a minimum average balance. The required amount is usually computed as a percentage of customer loans outstanding or as a percentage of the future loans to which the bank has committed itself.
Estate	An estate is the totality of the legal rights, interests, entitlements and obligations attaching to property. In the context of wills and probate, it refers to the totality of the property which the deceased owned or in which some interest was held.
Depository bank	The bank where the payee or holder has an account is referred to as a depository bank.
Mortgage bond	Type of secured bond that conditionally transfers title of a designated piece of property to the bondholder until the bond is paid is referred to as mortgage bond.
Mortgage	Mortgage refers to a note payable issued for property, such as a house, usually repaid in equal installments consisting of part principle and part interest, over a specified period.
Purchase order	A form on which items or services needed by a business firm are specified and then communicated to the vendor is a purchase order.
Average cost	Average cost is equal to total cost divided by the number of goods produced (Quantity-Q). It is also equal to the sum of average variable costs (total variable costs divided by Q) plus average fixed costs (total fixed costs divided by Q).
Treasury security	A treasury security is a government bond issued by the United States Department of the Treasury through the Bureau of the Public Debt. They are the debt financing instruments of the U.S. Federal government, and are often referred to simply as Treasuries.
Standing	Standing refers to the legal requirement that anyone seeking to challenge a particular action in court must demonstrate that such action substantially affects his legitimate interests before he will be entitled to bring suit.
Net trade credit	Net trade credit refers to a measure of the relationship between the firm's accounts receivable and accounts payable. If accounts receivable exceed accounts payable, the firm is a net provider of trade credit; otherwise, it is a net user.
Pledge	In law a pledge (also pawn) is a bailment of personal property as a security for some debt or engagement.
Control charts	Control charts refer to tools for monitoring process variation.
Control chart	The control chart, also known as the 'Shewhart chart' or 'process-behavior chart' is a statistical tool intended to assess the nature of variation in a process and to facilitate forecasting and management. The control chart is one of the seven basic tools of quality control, which include the histogram, Pareto chart, check sheet, control chart, cause-and-effect diagram, flowchart, and scatter diagram.
Investment management	Investment management is a branch of investment analysis that looks into the process of managing money. Investment portfolios can be managed through decisions about security purchases and sales.
Working capital	The dollar difference between total current assets and total current liabilities is called working capital.
Preference	The act of a debtor in paying or securing one or more of his creditors in a manner more favorable to them than to other creditors or to the exclusion of such other creditors is a

Chapter 16. Current Asset Management and Financing

Chapter 16. Current Asset Management and Financing

	preference. In the absence of statute, a preference is perfectly good, but to be legal it must be bona fide, and not a mere subterfuge of the debtor to secure a future benefit to himself or to prevent the application of his property to his debts.
Tactic	A short-term immediate decision that, in its totality, leads to the achievement of strategic goals is called a tactic.
Resource management	Resource management is the efficient and effective deployment of an organization's resources when they are needed. Such resources may include financial resources, inventory, human skills, production resources, or information technology.
Administration	Administration refers to the management and direction of the affairs of governments and institutions; a collective term for all policymaking officials of a government; the execution and implementation of public policy.
Vendor	A person who sells property to a vendee is a vendor. The words vendor and vendee are more commonly applied to the seller and purchaser of real estate, and the words seller and buyer are more commonly applied to the seller and purchaser of personal property.
Medicare	Medicare refers to federal program that is financed by payroll taxes and provides for compulsory hospital insurance for senior citizens and low-cost voluntary insurance to help older Americans pay physicians' fees.
Journal	Book of original entry, in which transactions are recorded in a general ledger system, is referred to as a journal.
Best practice	Best practice is a management idea which asserts that there is a technique, method, process, activity, incentive or reward that is more effective at delivering a particular outcome than any other technique, method, process, etc.
Option	A contract that gives the purchaser the option to buy or sell the underlying financial instrument at a specified price, called the exercise price or strike price, within a specific period of time.
Securitization	Securitization is a financing technique that allows the corporation to separate credit origination and funding activities. The technique comes under the umbrella of structured finance as it applies to assets that typically are illiquid contracts.

Chapter 16. Current Asset Management and Financing

Chapter 17. Analyzing Financial Performance

Financial statement	Financial statement refers to a summary of all the transactions that have occurred over a particular period.
Economic value added	After-tax operating income minus the weighted average cost of capital multiplied by total assets minus current liabilities is called economic value added.
Market value added	Market value added is the difference between the current market value of a firm and the capital contributed by investors. If market value added is positive, the firm has added value. If it is negative the firm has destroyed value.
Market value	Market value refers to the price of an asset agreed on between a willing buyer and a willing seller; the price an asset could demand if it is sold on the open market.
Value added	The value of output minus the value of all intermediate inputs, representing therefore the contribution of, and payments to, primary factors of production a value added.
Market	A market is, as defined in economics, a social arrangement that allows buyers and sellers to discover information and carry out a voluntary exchange of goods or services.
Productivity	Productivity refers to the total output of goods and services in a given period of time divided by work hours.
Operation	A standardized method or technique that is performed repetitively, often on different materials resulting in different finished goods is called an operation.
Service	Service refers to a "non tangible product" that is not embodied in a physical good and that typically effects some change in another product, person, or institution. Contrasts with good.
Liability	A liability is a present obligation of the enterprise arizing from past events, the settlement of which is expected to result in an outflow from the enterprise of resources embodying economic benefits.
Firm	An organization that employs resources to produce a good or service for profit and owns and operates one or more plants is referred to as a firm.
Bleed	Printed matter that runs over the edges of an outdoor board or of a page, leaving no margin is called a bleed.
Investing activities	Investing activities refers to cash flow activities that include purchasing and disposing of investments and productive long-lived assets using cash and lending money and collecting on those loans.
Fixed asset	Fixed asset, also known as property, plant, and equipment (PP&E), is a term used in accountancy for assets and property which cannot easily be converted into cash. This can be compared with current assets such as cash or bank accounts, which are described as liquid assets. In most cases, only tangible assets are referred to as fixed.
Cash flow	In finance, cash flow refers to the amounts of cash being received and spent by a business during a defined period of time, sometimes tied to a specific project. Most of the time they are being used to determine gaps in the liquid position of a company.
Asset	An item of property, such as land, capital, money, a share in ownership, or a claim on others for future payment, such as a bond or a bank deposit is an asset.
Statement of cash flow	Reports inflows and outflows of cash during the accounting period in the categories of operating, investing, and financing is a statement of cash flow.
Income statement	Income statement refers to a financial statement that presents the revenues and expenses and resulting net income or net loss of a company for a specific period of time.
Ratio analysis	Ratio analysis refers to an analytical tool designed to identify significant relationships;

Chapter 17. Analyzing Financial Performance

Chapter 17. Analyzing Financial Performance

	measures the proportional relationship between two financial statement amounts.
Balance sheet	A statement of the assets, liabilities, and net worth of a firm or individual at some given time often at the end of its "fiscal year," is referred to as a balance sheet.
Balance	In banking and accountancy, the outstanding balance is the amount of money owned, (or due), that remains in a deposit account (or a loan account) at a given date, after all past remittances, payments and withdrawal have been accounted for. It can be positive (then, in the balance sheet of a firm, it is an asset) or negative (a liability).
Principal	In agency law, one under whose direction an agent acts and for whose benefit that agent acts is a principal.
Interest	In finance and economics, interest is the price paid by a borrower for the use of a lender's money. In other words, interest is the amount of paid to "rent" money for a period of time.
Financial ratio	A financial ratio is a ratio of two numbers of reported levels or flows of a company. It may be two financial flows categories divided by each other (profit margin, profit/revenue). It may be a level divided by a financial flow (price/earnings). It may be a flow divided by a level (return on equity or earnings/equity). The numerator or denominator may itself be a ratio (PEG ratio).
Industry	A group of firms that produce identical or similar products is an industry. It is also used specifically to refer to an area of economic production focused on manufacturing which involves large amounts of capital investment before any profit can be realized, also called "heavy industry".
Profitability ratios	Measures of the income or operating success of a company for a given period of time are called profitability ratios.
Profitability ratio	A financial ratio that describes the firm's profits is referred to as profitability ratio. It helps to explain the profitability of an entity during a defined period of time.
Policy	Similar to a script in that a policy can be a less than completely rational decision-making method. Involves the use of a pre-existing set of decision steps for any problem that presents itself.
Profit margin	Profit margin is a measure of profitability. It is calculated using a formula and written as a percentage or a number. Profit margin = Net income before tax and interest / Revenue.
Total revenue	Total revenue refers to the total number of dollars received by a firm from the sale of a product; equal to the total expenditures for the product produced by the firm; equal to the quantity sold multiplied by the price at which it is sold.
Net income	Net income is equal to the income that a firm has after subtracting costs and expenses from the total revenue. Expenses will typically include tax expense.
Revenue	Revenue is a U.S. business term for the amount of money that a company receives from its activities, mostly from sales of products and/or services to customers.
Profit	Profit refers to the return to the resource entrepreneurial ability; total revenue minus total cost.
Margin	A deposit by a buyer in stocks with a seller or a stockbroker, as security to cover fluctuations in the market in reference to stocks that the buyer has purchased but for which he has not paid is a margin. Commodities are also traded on margin.
Expense	In accounting, an expense represents an event in which an asset is used up or a liability is incurred. In terms of the accounting equation, expenses reduce owners' equity.
Quartile	A quartile is any of the three values which divides sorted data set into four equal parts, so

Chapter 17. Analyzing Financial Performance

Chapter 17. Analyzing Financial Performance

	that each part represents 1/4th of the sample or population.
Allowance	Reduction in the selling price of goods extended to the buyer because the goods are defective or of lower quality than the buyer ordered and to encourage a buyer to keep merchandise that would otherwise be returned is the allowance.
Operating margin	In business, operating margin is the ratio of operating income divided by net sales.
Operating income	Total revenues from operation minus cost of goods sold and operating costs are called operating income.
Business operations	Business operations are those activities involved in the running of a business for the purpose of producing value for the stakeholders. The outcome of business operations is the harvesting of value from assets owned by a business.
Core business	The core business of an organization is an idealized construct intended to express that organization's "main" or "essential" activity.
Core	A core is the set of feasible allocations in an economy that cannot be improved upon by subset of the set of the economy's consumers (a coalition). In construction, when the force in an element is within a certain center section, the core, the element will only be under compression.
Gain	In finance, gain is a profit or an increase in value of an investment such as a stock or bond. Gain is calculated by fair market value or the proceeds from the sale of the investment minus the sum of the purchase price and all costs associated with it.
Return on Assets	The Return on Assets percentage shows how profitable a company's assets are in generating revenue.
Return on equity	Net profit after taxes per dollar of equity capital is referred to as return on equity.
Net assets	Net assets refers to portion of the assets remaining after the creditors' claims have been satisfied; also called equity or residual interest.
Equity	Equity is the name given to the set of legal principles, in countries following the English common law tradition, which supplement strict rules of law where their application would operate harshly, so as to achieve what is sometimes referred to as "natural justice."
Equity investment	Equity investment generally refers to the buying and holding of shares of stock on a stock market by individuals and funds in anticipation of income from dividends and capital gain as the value of the stock rises.
Investment	Investment refers to spending for the production and accumulation of capital and additions to inventories. In a financial sense, buying an asset with the expectation of making a return.
Capital	Capital generally refers to financial wealth, especially that used to start or maintain a business. In classical economics, capital is one of four factors of production, the others being land and labor and entrepreneurship.
Liquidity ratio	A financial ratio that indicates the organization's ability to meet its current debt obligations is referred to as liquidity ratio.
Liquidity	Liquidity refers to the capacity to turn assets into cash, or the amount of assets in a portfolio that have that capacity.
Creditor	A person to whom a debt or legal obligation is owed, and who has the right to enforce payment of that debt or obligation is referred to as creditor.
Current liability	Current liability refers to a debt that can reasonably be expected to be paid from existing current assets or through the creation of other current liabilities, within one year or the operating cycle, whichever is longer.

Go to **Cram101.com** for the Practice Tests for this Chapter.

Chapter 17. Analyzing Financial Performance

Chapter 17. Analyzing Financial Performance

Current ratio	The current ratio is a comparison of a firm's current assets to its current liabilities. The current ratio is an indication of a firm's market liquidity and ability to meet short-term debt obligations.
Current asset	A current asset is an asset on the balance sheet which is expected to be sold or otherwise used up in the near future, usually within one year.
Liquidation	Liquidation refers to a process whereby the assets of a business are converted to money. The conversion may be coerced by a legal process to pay off the debt of the business, or to satisfy any other business obligation that the business has not voluntarily satisfied.
Book value	The book value of an asset or group of assets is sometimes the price at which they were originally acquired, in many cases equal to purchase price.
Accounts payable	A written record of all vendors to whom the business firm owes money is referred to as accounts payable.
Notes payable	Notes payable refers to an obligation in the form of a written promissory note. It is a balance sheet term referring to a company's outstanding bank loans.
Stated value	An arbitrary dollar amount assigned to shares by the board of directors, representing the minimum amount of consideration for which the corporation may issue the shares and the portion of consideration that must be allocated to the stated capital account is the stated value.
Liquidated	Damages made certain by the prior agreement of the parties are called liquidated.
Depreciation	Depreciation is an accounting and finance term for the method of attributing the cost of an asset across the useful life of the asset. Depreciation is a reduction in the value of a currency in floating exchange rate.
Security	Security refers to a claim on the borrower future income that is sold by the borrower to the lender. A security is a type of transferable interest representing financial value.
Marketable securities	Marketable securities refer to securities that are readily traded in the secondary securities market.
Financial leverage	A measure of the amount of debt used in the capital structure of the firm is the financial leverage.
Capital structure	Capital Structure refers to the way a corporation finances itself through some combination of equity sales, equity options, bonds, and loans. Optimal capital structure refers to the particular combination that minimizes the cost of capital while maximizing the stock price.
Debt financing	Obtaining financing by borrowing money is debt financing.
Management	Management characterizes the process of leading and directing all or part of an organization, often a business, through the deployment and manipulation of resources. Early twentieth-century management writer Mary Parker Follett defined management as "the art of getting things done through people."
Leverage	Leverage is using given resources in such a way that the potential positive or negative outcome is magnified. In finance, this generally refers to borrowing.
Capital lease	A type of lease whose characteristics make it similar to a debt-financed purchase and that is consequently accounted for in that fashion is called capital lease. A capital lease is usually used to finance equipment for the major part of its useful life, and there is a reasonable assurance that the lessee will obtain ownership of the equipment by the end of the lease term.
Debt ratio	Debt ratio refers to the calculation of the total liabilities divided by the total

Chapter 17. Analyzing Financial Performance

Chapter 17. Analyzing Financial Performance

	liabilities plus capital. This results in the measurment of the debt level of the business (leverage).
Lease	A contract for the possession and use of land or other property, including goods, on one side, and a recompense of rent or other income on the other is the lease.
Bankruptcy	Bankruptcy is a legally declared inability or impairment of ability of an individual or organization to pay their creditors.
Fund	Independent accounting entity with a self-balancing set of accounts segregated for the purposes of carrying on specific activities is referred to as a fund.
Equity capital	Equity capital refers to money raized from within the firm or through the sale of ownership in the firm.
Debt to equity ratio	The debt to equity ratio is a financial ratio debt divided by shareholders' equity. The two components are often taken from the firm's balance sheet, but they might also be calulated as market values if both the companiy's debt and equity are publicly traded. It is used to calculate a company's "financial leverage" and indicates what proportion of equity and debt the company is using to finance its assets.
Lender	Suppliers and financial institutions that lend money to companies is referred to as a lender.
Times interest earned	Times interest earned refers to net income before interest and taxes, divided by interest expense; describes a company's ability to make interest payments on its debt.
Accounting income	The accountant's concept of income is generally based upon the realization principle. Financial accounting income may differ from taxable income. Differences are included in a reconciliation of taxable and accounting income on Schedule M-1 of Form 1120.
Interest expense	The cost a business incurs to borrow money. With respect to bonds payable, the interest expense is calculated by multiplying the market rate of interest by the carrying value of the bonds on the date of the payment.
Accounting	A system that collects and processes financial information about an organization and reports that information to decision makers is referred to as accounting.
Margin of safety	Margin of safety is the difference between the intrinsic value of a stock (i.e. value based on stock valuation and what the company is actually worth) and the price that the market sets on a stock (i.e. stock price is a matter of market participants' opinions and is different from the intrinsic value).
Asset management	Asset management is the method that a company uses to track fixed assets, for example factory equipment, desks and chairs, computers, even buildings. Although the exact details of the task varies widely from company to company, asset management often includes tracking the physical location of assets, managing demand for scarce resources, and accounting tasks such as amortization.
Asset turnover ratio	A measure of how efficiently a company uses its assets to generate sales, an asset turnover ratio is computed as net sales divided by average total assets.
Turnover	Turnover in a financial context refers to the rate at which a provider of goods cycles through its average inventory. Turnover in a human resources context refers to the characteristic of a given company or industry, relative to rate at which an employer gains and loses staff.
Historical cost	In accounting terminology, historical cost describes the original cost of an asset at the time of purchase or payment as opposed to its market value
Inflation	An increase in the overall price level of an economy, usually as measured by the CPI or by the implicit price deflator is called inflation.

Go to Cram101.com for the Practice Tests for this Chapter.

Chapter 17. Analyzing Financial Performance

Chapter 17. Analyzing Financial Performance

Accounts receivable	Accounts receivable is one of a series of accounting transactions dealing with the billing of customers which owe money to a person, company or organization for goods and services that have been provided to the customer. This is typically done in a one person organization by writing an invoice and mailing or delivering it to each customer.
Premium	Premium refers to the fee charged by an insurance company for an insurance policy. The rate of losses must be relatively predictable: In order to set the premium (prices) insurers must be able to estimate them accurately.
Accumulated depreciation	Accumulated depreciation refers to the total depreciation that has been reported as depreciation expense for the entire life of a long-term tangible asset. It is a contra-asset account.
Depreciation expense	Depreciation expense refers to the amount recognized as an expense in one period resulting from the periodic recognition of the used portion of the cost of a long-term tangible asset over its life.
Physical asset	A physical asset is an item of economic value that has a tangible or material existence. A physical asset usually refers to cash, equipment, inventory and properties owned by a business.
Book value per share	Total shareholders' equity divided by the number of outstanding common shares is referred to as book value per share.
Stock	In financial terminology, stock is the capital raized by a corporation, through the issuance and sale of shares.
P/E ratio	In finance, the P/E ratio of a stock is used to measure how cheap or expensive share prices are. It is probably the single most consistent red flag to excessive optimism and over-investment.
Market price	Market price is an economic concept with commonplace familiarity; it is the price that a good or service is offered at, or will fetch, in the marketplace; it is of interest mainly in the study of microeconomics.
Shares	Shares refer to an equity security, representing a shareholder's ownership of a corporation. Shares are one of a finite number of equal portions in the capital of a company, entitling the owner to a proportion of distributed, non-reinvested profits known as dividends and to a portion of the value of the company in case of liquidation.
Trend analysis	A comparison across time of three or more observations of a particular financial item, such as net income, is called trend analysis.
Trend	Trend refers to the long-term movement of an economic variable, such as its average rate of increase or decrease over enough years to encompass several business cycles.
Holding	The holding is a court's determination of a matter of law based on the issue presented in the particular case. In other words: under this law, with these facts, this result.
Tying	Tying is the practice of making the sale of one good (the tying good) to the de facto or de jure customer conditional on the purchase of a second distinctive good.
Equity multiplier	The amount of assets per dollar of equity capital is referred to as equity multiplier.
Equity financing	Financing that consists of funds that are invested in exchange for ownership in the company is called equity financing.
Marketing	Promoting and selling products or services to customers, or prospective customers, is referred to as marketing.

Chapter 17. Analyzing Financial Performance

Chapter 17. Analyzing Financial Performance

Analyst	Analyst refers to a person or tool with a primary function of information analysis, generally with a more limited, practical and short term set of goals than a researcher.
Variable	A variable is something measured by a number; it is used to analyze what happens to other things when the size of that number changes.
Shareholder wealth maximization	Shareholder wealth maximization refers to maximizing the wealth of the firm's shareholders through achieving the highest possible value for the firm in the marketplace. It is the overriding objective of the firm and should influence all decisions.
Shareholder	A shareholder is an individual or company (including a corporation) that legally owns one or more shares of stock in a joined stock company.
Frequency	Frequency refers to the speed of the up and down movements of a fluctuating economic variable; that is, the number of times per unit of time that the variable completes a cycle of up and down movement.
Time value of money	Time value of money is the concept that the value of money varies depending on the timing of the cash flows, given any interest rate greater than zero.
Value of money	Value of money refers to the quantity of goods and services for which a unit of money can be exchanged; the purchasing power of a unit of money; the reciprocal of the price level.
Contribution	In business organization law, the cash or property contributed to a business by its owners is referred to as contribution.
Cost of capital	Cost of capital refers to the percentage cost of funds used for acquiring resources for an organization, typically a weighted average of the firms cost of equity and cost of debt.
Economic profit	In Economics, a firm is said to be making an economic profit when its revenue exceeds the total opportunity cost of its inputs. It is said to be making an accounting profit if its revenues exceed the total price the firm pays for those inputs. This is sometimes referred to as producer's surplus.
Residual	Residual payments can refer to an ongoing stream of payments in respect of the completion of past achievements.
Opportunity cost	The cost of something in terms of opportunity foregone. The opportunity cost to a country of producing a unit more of a good, such as for export or to replace an import, is the quantity of some other good that could have been produced instead.
Residual income	Residual income is the term used to describe income received based on the production of those others who have become members of one's organization.
Business unit	The lowest level of the company which contains the set of functions that carry a product through its life span from concept through manufacture, distribution, sales and service is a business unit.
Operating profit	Operating profit is a measure of a company's earning power from ongoing operations, equal to earnings before the deduction of interest payments and income taxes.
Amortization	Systematic and rational allocation of the acquisition cost of an intangible asset over its useful life is referred to as amortization.
Inventory	Tangible property held for sale in the normal course of business or used in producing goods or services for sale is an inventory.
Valuation	In finance, valuation is the process of estimating the market value of a financial asset or liability. They can be done on assets (for example, investments in marketable securities such as stocks, options, business enterprises, or intangible assets such as patents and trademarks) or on liabilities (e.g., Bonds issued by a company).

Go to **Cram101.com** for the Practice Tests for this Chapter.

Chapter 17. Analyzing Financial Performance

Chapter 17. Analyzing Financial Performance

Research and development	The use of resources for the deliberate discovery of new information and ways of doing things, together with the application of that information in inventing new products or processes is referred to as research and development.
Benchmarking	The continuous process of comparing the levels of performance in producing products and services and executing activities against the best levels of performance is benchmarking.
Evaluation	The consumer's appraisal of the product or brand on important attributes is called evaluation.
Competitor	Other organizations in the same industry or type of business that provide a good or service to the same set of customers is referred to as a competitor.
Average revenue	Average revenue refers to total revenue from the sale of a product divided by the quantity of the product sold ; equal to the price at which the product is sold when all units of the product are sold at the same price.
Bad debt	In accounting and finance, bad debt is the portion of receivables that can no longer be collected, typically from accounts receivable or loans. Bad debt in accounting is considered an expense.
Medicare	Medicare refers to federal program that is financed by payroll taxes and provides for compulsory hospital insurance for senior citizens and low-cost voluntary insurance to help older Americans pay physicians' fees.
Financial analysis	Financial analysis is the analysis of the accounts and the economic prospects of a firm.
Weighted average	The weighted average unit cost of the goods available for sale for both cost of goods sold and ending inventory.
Operating expense	In throughput accounting, the cost accounting aspect of Theory of Constraints (TOC), operating expense is the money spent turning inventory into throughput. In TOC, operating expense is limited to costs that vary strictly with the quantity produced, like raw materials and purchased components.
Distortion	Distortion refers to any departure from the ideal of perfect competition that interferes with economic agents maximizing social welfare when they maximize their own.
Rate of return	A rate of return is a comparison of the money earned (or lost) on an investment to the amount of money invested.
Operating cash flows	Operating cash flows refers to the cash inflows and cash outflows from the general operating activities of the business; one of the three sections in the statement of cash flows.
Debt service	The payments made by a borrower on their debt, usually including both interest payments and partial repayment of principal, are called debt service.
Operating results	Operating results refers to measures that are important to monitoring and tracking the effectiveness of a company's operations.
Inventory turnover ratio	Inventory turnover ratio refers to a ratio that measures the number of times on average the inventory sold during the period; computed by dividing cost of goods sold by the average inventory during the period.
Fiscal year	A fiscal year is a 12-month period used for calculating annual ("yearly") financial reports in businesses and other organizations. In many jurisdictions, regulatory laws regarding accounting require such reports once per twelve months, but do not require that the twelve months constitute a calendar year (i.e. January to December).
Enterprise	Enterprise refers to another name for a business organization. Other similar terms are

Chapter 17. Analyzing Financial Performance

Chapter 17. Analyzing Financial Performance

	business firm, sometimes simply business, sometimes simply firm, as well as company, and entity.
Current account	Current account refers to a country's international transactions arising from current flows, as opposed to changes in stocks which are part of the capital account. Includes trade in goods and services plus inflows and outflows of transfers. A current account is a deposit account in the UK and countries with a UK banking heritage.
Credit	Credit refers to a recording as positive in the balance of payments, any transaction that gives rise to a payment into the country, such as an export, the sale of an asset, or borrowing from abroad.
Retained earnings	Cumulative earnings of a company that are not distributed to the owners and are reinvested in the business are called retained earnings.
Insurance	Insurance refers to a system by which individuals can reduce their exposure to risk of large losses by spreading the risks among a large number of persons.
Supply	Supply is the aggregate amount of any material good that can be called into being at a certain price point; it comprises one half of the equation of supply and demand. In classical economic theory, a curve representing supply is one of the factors that produce price.
Common stock	Common stock refers to the basic, normal, voting stock issued by a corporation; called residual equity because it ranks after preferred stock for dividend and liquidation distributions.
Property	Assets defined in the broadest legal sense. Property includes the unrealized receivables of a cash basis taxpayer, but not services rendered.
Credit sale	A credit sale occurs when a customer does not pay cash at the time of the sale but instead agrees to pay later. The sale occurs now, with payment from the customer to follow at a later time.
Insolvency	Insolvency is a financial condition experienced by a person or business entity when their assets no longer exceed their liabilities or when the person or entity can no longer meet its debt obligations when they come due.
Journal	Book of original entry, in which transactions are recorded in a general ledger system, is referred to as a journal.
Financial management	The job of managing a firm's resources so it can meet its goals and objectives is called financial management.
Administration	Administration refers to the management and direction of the affairs of governments and institutions; a collective term for all policymaking officials of a government; the execution and implementation of public policy.
Financial distress	Financial distress is a term in Corporate Finance used to indicate a condition when promises to creditors of a company are broken or honored with difficulty. Sometimes financial distress can lead to bankruptcy. Financial distress is usually associated with some costs to the company and these are known as Costs of Financial Distress. A common example of a cost of financial distress is bankrupty costs.
Balanced scorecard	A framework for implementing strategy by translating an organization's mission and strategy into a set of performance measures is called balanced scorecard.
Creditworthiness	Creditworthiness indicates whether a borrower has in the past made loan payments when due.
Performance measurement	The process by which someone evaluates an employee's work behaviors by measurement and comparison with previously established standards, documents the results, and communicates the results to the employee is called performance measurement.

Chapter 17. Analyzing Financial Performance

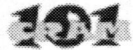

Go to **Cram101.com** for the Practice Tests for this Chapter.

Chapter 17. Analyzing Financial Performance

Chapter 18. Lease Financing and Business Valuation

Lessee	One who rents property from another. In the case of real estate, the lessee is also known as the tenant.
Lease	A contract for the possession and use of land or other property, including goods, on one side, and a recompense of rent or other income on the other is the lease.
Discounted cash flow	In finance, the discounted cash flow approach describes a method to value a project or an entire company. The DCF methods determine the present value of future cash flows by discounting them using the appropriate cost of capital.
Valuation	In finance, valuation is the process of estimating the market value of a financial asset or liability. They can be done on assets (for example, investments in marketable securities such as stocks, options, business enterprises, or intangible assets such as patents and trademarks) or on liabilities (e.g., Bonds issued by a company).
Cash flow	In finance, cash flow refers to the amounts of cash being received and spent by a business during a defined period of time, sometimes tied to a specific project. Most of the time they are being used to determine gaps in the liquid position of a company.
Market	A market is, as defined in economics, a social arrangement that allows buyers and sellers to discover information and carry out a voluntary exchange of goods or services.
Debt financing	Obtaining financing by borrowing money is debt financing.
Acquisition	A company's purchase of the property and obligations of another company is an acquisition.
Capital	Capital generally refers to financial wealth, especially that used to start or maintain a business. In classical economics, capital is one of four factors of production, the others being land and labor and entrepreneurship.
Merger	Merger refers to the combination of two firms into a single firm.
Fixed asset	Fixed asset, also known as property, plant, and equipment (PP&E), is a term used in accountancy for assets and property which cannot easily be converted into cash. This can be compared with current assets such as cash or bank accounts, which are described as liquid assets. In most cases, only tangible assets are referred to as fixed.
Asset	An item of property, such as land, capital, money, a share in ownership, or a claim on others for future payment, such as a bond or a bank deposit is an asset.
Equity capital	Equity capital refers to money raized from within the firm or through the sale of ownership in the firm.
Equity	Equity is the name given to the set of legal principles, in countries following the English common law tradition, which supplement strict rules of law where their application would operate harshly, so as to achieve what is sometimes referred to as "natural justice."
Estate	An estate is the totality of the legal rights, interests, entitlements and obligations attaching to property. In the context of wills and probate, it refers to the totality of the property which the deceased owned or in which some interest was held.
Technology	The body of knowledge and techniques that can be used to combine economic resources to produce goods and services is called technology.
Industry	A group of firms that produce identical or similar products is an industry. It is also used specifically to refer to an area of economic production focused on manufacturing which involves large amounts of capital investment before any profit can be realized, also called "heavy industry".
Service	Service refers to a "non tangible product" that is not embodied in a physical good and that typically effects some change in another product, person, or institution. Contrasts with

Chapter 18. Lease Financing and Business Valuation

Chapter 18. Lease Financing and Business Valuation

		good.
Information technology		Information technology refers to technology that helps companies change business by allowing them to use new methods.
Property		Assets defined in the broadest legal sense. Property includes the unrealized receivables of a cash basis taxpayer, but not services rendered.
Lessor		The person who transfers the right of possession and use of goods under the lease is referred to as lessor.
Operating lease		Operating lease refers to a contractual arrangement giving the lessee temporary use of the property with continued ownership of the property by the lessor. Accounted for as a rental.
Financial lease		A long-term, non-cancelable lease is a financial lease. The financial lease has all the characteristics of long-term debt.
Contract		A contract is a "promise" or an "agreement" that is enforced or recognized by the law. In the civil law, a contract is considered to be part of the general law of obligations.
Useful life		The length of service of a productive facility or piece of equipment is its useful life. The period of time during which an asset will have economic value and be usable.
Rate of return		A rate of return is a comparison of the money earned (or lost) on an investment to the amount of money invested.
Amortization		Systematic and rational allocation of the acquisition cost of an intangible asset over its useful life is referred to as amortization.
Investment		Investment refers to spending for the production and accumulation of capital and additions to inventories. In a financial sense, buying an asset with the expectation of making a return.
Term loan		Term loan refers to an intermediate-length loan, in which credit is generally extended from one to seven years. The loan is usually repaid in monthly or quarterly installments over its life, rather than with one single payment.
Secured loan		Secured loan refers to a loan backed by something valuable, such as property.
Amortize		To provide for the payment of a debt by creating a sinking fund or paying in installments is to amortize.
Balance		In banking and accountancy, the outstanding balance is the amount of money owned, (or due), that remains in a deposit account (or a loan account) at a given date, after all past remittances, payments and withdrawal have been accounted for. It can be positive (then, in the balance sheet of a firm, it is an asset) or negative (a liability).
Lender		Suppliers and financial institutions that lend money to companies is referred to as a lender.
Exchange		The trade of things of value between buyer and seller so that each is better off after the trade is called the exchange.
Expense		In accounting, an expense represents an event in which an asset is used up or a liability is incurred. In terms of the accounting equation, expenses reduce owners' equity.
Depreciation		Depreciation is an accounting and finance term for the method of attributing the cost of an asset across the useful life of the asset. Depreciation is a reduction in the value of a currency in floating exchange rate.
Deductible		The dollar sum of costs that an insured individual must pay before the insurer begins to pay is called deductible.
Finance lease		A three-party transaction consisting of the lessor, the lessee, and the supplier is referred to as the finance lease.

Chapter 18. Lease Financing and Business Valuation

Chapter 18. Lease Financing and Business Valuation

Depreciate	A nation's currency is said to depreciate when exchange rates change so that a unit of its currency can buy fewer units of foreign currency.
Firm	An organization that employs resources to produce a good or service for profit and owns and operates one or more plants is referred to as a firm.
Financial transaction	A financial transaction involves a change in the status of the finances of two or more businesses or individuals.
Interest	In finance and economics, interest is the price paid by a borrower for the use of a lender's money. In other words, interest is the amount of paid to "rent" money for a period of time.
Present value	The value today of a stream of payments and/or receipts over time in the future and/or the past, converted to the present using an interest rate. If X_t is the amount in period t and r the interest rate, then present value at time t=0 is $V = ?T /t$.
Balance sheet	A statement of the assets, liabilities, and net worth of a firm or individual at some given time often at the end of its "fiscal year," is referred to as a balance sheet.
Liability	A liability is a present obligation of the enterprise arizing from past events, the settlement of which is expected to result in an outflow from the enterprise of resources embodying economic benefits.
Bankruptcy	Bankruptcy is a legally declared inability or impairment of ability of an individual or organization to pay their creditors.
Debt ratio	Debt ratio refers to the calculation of the total liabilities divided by the total liabilities plus capital. This results in the measurment of the debt level of the business (leverage).
Accounting	A system that collects and processes financial information about an organization and reports that information to decision makers is referred to as accounting.
Interest payment	The payment to holders of bonds payable, calculated by multiplying the stated rate on the face of the bond by the par, or face, value of the bond. If bonds are issued at a discount or premium, the interest payment does not equal the interest expense.
Capital lease	A type of lease whose characteristics make it similar to a debt-financed purchase and that is consequently accounted for in that fashion is called capital lease. A capital lease is usually used to finance equipment for the major part of its useful life, and there is a reasonable assurance that the lessee will obtain ownership of the equipment by the end of the lease term.
Principal	In agency law, one under whose direction an agent acts and for whose benefit that agent acts is a principal.
Financial distress	Financial distress is a term in Corporate Finance used to indicate a condition when promises to creditors of a company are broken or honored with difficulty. Sometimes financial distress can lead to bankruptcy. Financial distress is usually associated with some costs to the company and these are known as Costs of Financial Distress. A common example of a cost of financial distress is bankrupty costs.
Market value	Market value refers to the price of an asset agreed on between a willing buyer and a willing seller; the price an asset could demand if it is sold on the open market.
Collateral	Property that is pledged to the lender to guarantee payment in the event that the borrower is unable to make debt payments is called collateral.
Closing	The finalization of a real estate sales transaction that passes title to the property from the seller to the buyer is referred to as a closing. Closing is a sales term which refers to the process of making a sale. It refers to reaching the final step, which may be an exchange

Go to **Cram101.com** for the Practice Tests for this Chapter.

Chapter 18. Lease Financing and Business Valuation

Chapter 18. Lease Financing and Business Valuation

	of money or acquiring a signature.
Evaluation	The consumer's appraisal of the product or brand on important attributes is called evaluation.
Aid	Assistance provided by countries and by international institutions such as the World Bank to developing countries in the form of monetary grants, loans at low interest rates, in kind, or a combination of these is called aid. Aid can also refer to assistance of any type rendered to benefit some group or individual.
Opportunity cost	The cost of something in terms of opportunity foregone. The opportunity cost to a country of producing a unit more of a good, such as for export or to replace an import, is the quantity of some other good that could have been produced instead.
Fund	Independent accounting entity with a self-balancing set of accounts segregated for the purposes of carrying on specific activities is referred to as a fund.
Simple interest	Simple interest is interest that accrues linearly. In other words, it grows by a certain fraction of the principal per time period.
Cost of debt	The cost of debt is the cost of borrowing money (usually denoted by Kd). It is derived by dividing debt's interest payments on the total market value of the debts.
Discount	The difference between the face value of a bond and its selling price, when a bond is sold for less than its face value it's referred to as a discount.
Discount rate	Discount rate refers to the rate, per year, at which future values are diminished to make them comparable to values in the present. Can be either subjective or objective.
Residual	Residual payments can refer to an ongoing stream of payments in respect of the completion of past achievements.
Residual value	Residual value is one of the constituents of a leasing calculus or operation. It describes the future value of a good in terms of percentage of depreciation of its initial value.
Marginal tax rate	The percentage of an additional dollar of earnings that goes to taxes is referred to as the marginal tax rate.
Depreciation expense	Depreciation expense refers to the amount recognized as an expense in one period resulting from the periodic recognition of the used portion of the cost of a long-term tangible asset over its life.
Allowance	Reduction in the selling price of goods extended to the buyer because the goods are defective or of lower quality than the buyer ordered and to encourage a buyer to keep merchandise that would otherwise be returned is the allowance.
Operation	A standardized method or technique that is performed repetitively, often on different materials resulting in different finished goods is called an operation.
Stock	In financial terminology, stock is the capital raised by a corporation, through the issuance and sale of shares.
Contract A	Contract A is a concept applied in Canadian contract law (a Common Law system country) which has recently been applied by courts regarding the fairness and equal treatment of bidders in a contract tendering process. Essentially this concept formalises previously applied precedents and strengthens the protection afforded to Contractors in the tendering process.
Management	Management characterizes the process of leading and directing all or part of an organization, often a business, through the deployment and manipulation of resources. Early twentieth-century management writer Mary Parker Follett defined management as "the art of getting things done through people."

Go to **Cram101.com** for the Practice Tests for this Chapter.

Chapter 18. Lease Financing and Business Valuation

Chapter 18. Lease Financing and Business Valuation

Economics	The social science dealing with the use of scarce resources to obtain the maximum satisfaction of society's virtually unlimited economic wants is an economics.
Cash outflow	Cash flowing out of the business from all sources over a period of time is cash outflow.
Points	Loan origination fees that may be deductible as interest by a buyer of property. A seller of property who pays points reduces the selling price by the amount of the points paid for the buyer.
Inputs	The inputs used by a firm or an economy are the labor, raw materials, electricity and other resources it uses to produce its outputs.
Tax shelters	Tax shelters refer to the typical tax shelter generated large losses in the early years of the activity. Investors would offset these losses against other types of income and, therefore, avoid paying income taxes on this income.
Stockholder	A stockholder is an individual or company (including a corporation) that legally owns one or more shares of stock in a joined stock company. The shareholders are the owners of a corporation. Companies listed at the stock market strive to enhance shareholder value.
Corporation	A legal entity chartered by a state or the Federal government that is distinct and separate from the individuals who own it is a corporation. This separation gives the corporation unique powers which other legal entities lack.
Accelerated depreciation	Methods that result in higher depreciation expense in the early years of an asset's life, and lower expense in the later years are referred to as accelerated depreciation.
Shareholder	A shareholder is an individual or company (including a corporation) that legally owns one or more shares of stock in a joined stock company.
Profit	Profit refers to the return to the resource entrepreneurial ability; total revenue minus total cost.
Diversification	Investing in a collection of assets whose returns do not always move together, with the result that overall risk is lower than for individual assets is referred to as diversification.
Purchasing	Purchasing refers to the function in a firm that searches for quality material resources, finds the best suppliers, and negotiates the best price for goods and services.
Portfolio	In finance, a portfolio is a collection of investments held by an institution or a private individual. Holding but not always a portfolio is part of an investment and risk-limiting strategy called diversification. By owning several assets, certain types of risk (in particular specific risk) can be reduced.
Risk premium	In finance, the risk premium can be the expected rate of return above the risk-free interest rate.
Premium	Premium refers to the fee charged by an insurance company for an insurance policy. The rate of losses must be relatively predictable: In order to set the premium (prices) insurers must be able to estimate them accurately.
Users	Users refer to people in the organization who actually use the product or service purchased by the buying center.
Incremental cost	Additional total cost incurred for an activity is called incremental cost. A form of costing that classifies costs into their fixed and variable elements in order to calculate the extra cost of making and selling an additional batch of units.
Option	A contract that gives the purchaser the option to buy or sell the underlying financial instrument at a specified price, called the exercise price or strike price, within a specific

Go to Cram101.com for the Practice Tests for this Chapter.

Chapter 18. Lease Financing and Business Valuation

Chapter 18. Lease Financing and Business Valuation

	period of time.
Credit risk	The risk of loss due to a counterparty defaulting on a contract, or more generally the risk of loss due to some "credit event" is called credit risk.
Credit	Credit refers to a recording as positive in the balance of payments, any transaction that gives rise to a payment into the country, such as an export, the sale of an asset, or borrowing from abroad.
Assessment	Collecting information and providing feedback to employees about their behavior, communication style, or skills is an assessment.
Buyout	A buyout is an investment transaction by which the entire or a controlling part of the stock of a company is sold. A firm buysout the stake of the company to strengthen its influence on the company's decision making body. A buyout can take the forms of a leveraged buyout or a management buyout.
Capital budgeting	Capital budgeting is the planning process used to determine a firm's long term investments such as new machinery, replacement machinery, new plants, new products, and research and development projects.
Cash flow forecast	Forecast that predicts the cash inflows and outflows in future periods is a cash flow forecast. It is a company's projected cash receipts and disbursements over a set time horizon.
Earnings before interest and taxes	Income from operations before subtracting interest expense and income taxes is an earnings before interest and taxes.
Subsidiary	A company that is controlled by another company or corporation is a subsidiary.
Revenue	Revenue is a U.S. business term for the amount of money that a company receives from its activities, mostly from sales of products and/or services to customers.
Cost of equity	In finance, the cost of equity is the minimum rate of return a firm must offer shareholders to compensate for waiting for their returns, and for bearing some risk.
Cost of capital	Cost of capital refers to the percentage cost of funds used for acquiring resources for an organization, typically a weighted average of the firms cost of equity and cost of debt.
Broker	In commerce, a broker is a party that mediates between a buyer and a seller. A broker who also acts as a seller or as a buyer becomes a principal party to the deal.
Shares	Shares refer to an equity security, representing a shareholder's ownership of a corporation. Shares are one of a finite number of equal portions in the capital of a company, entitling the owner to a proportion of distributed, non-reinvested profits known as dividends and to a portion of the value of the company in case of liquidation.
Net profit	Net profit is an accounting term which is commonly used in business. It is equal to the gross revenue for a given time period minus associated expenses.
Operating cash flows	Operating cash flows refers to the cash inflows and cash outflows from the general operating activities of the business; one of the three sections in the statement of cash flows.
Terminal value	In finance, the terminal value of a security is the present value at a future point in time of all future cash flows. It is most often used in multi-stage discounted cash flow analysis, and allows for the limitation of cash flow projections to a several-year period.
Scenario analysis	Scenario analysis is a process of analyzing possible future events by considering alternative possible outcomes. The analysis is designed to allow improved decision-making by allowing more complete consideration of outcomes and their implications.
Proxy	Proxy refers to a person who is authorized to vote the shares of another person. Also, the

Chapter 18. Lease Financing and Business Valuation

Chapter 18. Lease Financing and Business Valuation

	written authorization empowering a person to vote the shares of another person.
Ad hoc	Ad hoc is a Latin phrase which means "for this purpose." It generally signifies a solution that has been tailored to a specific purpose and is makeshift and non-general, such as a handcrafted network protocol or a specific-purpose equation, as opposed to general solutions.
Comparability	Ability to compare the accounting information of different companies because they use the same accounting principles is known as comparability.
Notes to the financial statements	Notes that clarify information presented in the financial statements, as well as expand upon it where additional detail is needed are notes to the financial statements.
Financial statement	Financial statement refers to a summary of all the transactions that have occurred over a particular period.
Rate differential	The controversial practice of newspapers charging significantly higher rates to national advertisers as compared to local accounts is called rate differential.
Liquidity	Liquidity refers to the capacity to turn assets into cash, or the amount of assets in a portfolio that have that capacity.
Interest rate	The rate of return on bonds, loans, or deposits. When one speaks of 'the' interest rate, it is usually in a model where there is only one.
Brand	A name, symbol, or design that identifies the goods or services of one seller or group of sellers and distinguishes them from the goods and services of competitors is a brand.
Exempt	Employees who are not covered by the Fair Labor Standards Act are exempt. Exempt employees are not eligible for overtime pay.
Asset management	Asset management is the method that a company uses to track fixed assets, for example factory equipment, desks and chairs, computers, even buildings. Although the exact details of the task varies widely from company to company, asset management often includes tracking the physical location of assets, managing demand for scarce resources, and accounting tasks such as amortization.
Financial management	The job of managing a firm's resources so it can meet its goals and objectives is called financial management.
Grant	Grant refers to an intergovernmental transfer of funds. Since the New Deal, state and local governments have become increasingly dependent upon federal grants for an almost infinite variety of programs.
Journal	Book of original entry, in which transactions are recorded in a general ledger system, is referred to as a journal.
Ambulatory surgery	Surgery done in the doctor's office or at a surgical center, and not requiring an overnight stay. Ambulatory surgery is general planned ahead of time. Maybe referred to as one-day, in-and-out, or outpatient surgery.
Intangible assets	Assets that have special rights but not physical substance are referred to as intangible assets.
Intangible asset	An intangible assets is defined as an asset that is not physical in nature. The most common types are trade secrets (e.g., customer lists and know-how), copyrights, patents, trademarks, and goodwill.
Administration	Administration refers to the management and direction of the affairs of governments and institutions; a collective term for all policymaking officials of a government; the execution and implementation of public policy.

Go to **Cram101.com** for the Practice Tests for this Chapter.

Chapter 18. Lease Financing and Business Valuation

Chapter 18. Lease Financing and Business Valuation

Joint venture	Joint venture refers to an undertaking by two parties for a specific purpose and duration, taking any of several legal forms.

Chapter 18. Lease Financing and Business Valuation

Printed in the United States
205327BV00002B/12/A

9 781428 812871